Yoga In School

A Primer for Teachers and Parents

MICHELINE FLAK

JACQUES DE COULON

EDITIONS SATYANANDASHRAM
Paris, France

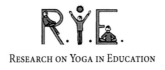

RESEARCH ON YOGA IN EDUCATION

*In gratefulness for the life of
Swami Satyananda, who instilled in us
the courage to sow the seeds of yoga
in the vast field of learning at school.*

*To our friends of RYE without whom
this book would not be what it is.
Many thanks also go to Michelle Blanquaert,
untiring secretary, and to Anne-Marie de Coulon
for her helpful advice.*

—The authors

*Many thanks to Mary Ann Baker,
whose unceasing work in favor of
yoga in education has made
this English version possible.*

—Micheline Flak

Table of Contents

Introduction

When yoga entered the classroom...

It began as a whispered rumor. Then it was spoken aloud. The clamor grew as the news spread. Ten years down the road, people still express surprise when they hear it:

"They're teaching yoga in the classroom! What's the world coming to?"

"Yoga, you say? But isn't that some sort of a sect or something?" ask the dumb-founded and uninformed.

"What do you mean yoga? How can they possibly expect children to practice postures in between chairs and tables? How can proper space be provided in classrooms?" ask those yogis who are wedded to their personal practice mats.

"Yoga! What in the world is that? Is it something new? Does it work?" asks a group of interested parents and teachers, who at least are willing to consider something new, provided it gives results.

Our experience of yoga in school, begun in 1973 at the College Condorcet, a middle school in Paris, France, has aroused a great deal of curiosity and interest as well as misunderstandings and misconceptions. It is easy to see why. The wide-spread fascination for yoga, as well as the current crisis in the world of education, is a manifestation of radical upheaval and change in our Western civilization. Introducing yoga practice at school leads us to reassess where we stand in education.

The alarming increase in the stress levels of our school children, and an exponential increase in the inability of children to pay attention, coincides with our own preference for natural remedies whenever possible.

We are writing here in answer to requests from numerous parents and teachers who recognize that our innovative method is an original and positive response to a very real concern: the health and success of the next generation.

Far too many children are tired, disconnected, hyperactive and unmotivated. We shouldn't necessarily give our own dysfunctional, adult solution as the example for them to follow. Neither should we expect the revolution in technology to replace the role of teachers in giving our children guidance in life skills.

We feel strongly that by teaching yoga in schools we can really help youngsters to adapt to the challenges of the twenty-first century.

This book is a mixture of simplicity and complexity. It delineates the basic principles of thought and scientific knowledge in the field of yoga applied to education.

Please allow us this amalgamation, which is a reflection of the principle of complementary opposites. We find examples of this in Oriental philosophy and cuisine, Chinese in particular, with its subtle combination of sugar and salt, tender and hard, red and green, black and white.

The seeming ease of the practical exercises presented here belies the many benefits to be reaped from them.

In every sense of the word, they are exercises which educate us in a new way of living and distill for us the quintessence of a good life.

PART ONE

THE LANDMARKS
OF SUCCESS

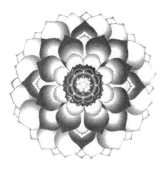

Sowing the Seeds of Yoga

It is the beginning of the school day. A group of fifth year pupils are piling into their classroom and opening their satchels. The usual pre-class commotion is in full swing. Books and folders are being opened noisily, pens and pencils rattling in their containers. Everything is ready for the lesson to start. The teacher begins to speak:

"Stand up, everyone! Today we are going to work with our whole bodies, not just our heads. We are going to practice 'being trees blowing in the wind'. First of all, feel yourselves rooted deeply in the ground. Then, when you are firmly planted, we shall do a balancing exercise. I'm not going to ask you to stand on one leg, so there is no need to grab hold of your tables or chairs. Just BE where you are, with both feet flat on the ground. Now stretch upwards, feeling the sensation in your whole body of standing straight and tall, just like a tree in the forest. You needn't shut your eyes just yet.

(There is total silence in the classroom.)

"Now, bear the entire weight of your body onto your right foot, still keeping your left foot on the floor. Now shift all your weight onto your left foot. Begin to sway, just like a tree balancing itself by moving from side to side, each to your own rhythm. Now sway backwards and forwards as the wind pushes you. Each of you is a tree in a forest full of trees. Feel the soles of your feet, anchoring you to the ground. Feel your strong trunk, swaying backwards and forwards and from side to side as you keep your balance against the wind. Listen to your branches crackling and sighing... Keep on swaying. You may want to close your eyes or fix your gaze on a point somewhere in front of you – whichever feels better for you."

(Pause, while the children experiment for themselves.)

3

"You can pretend to be the wind, as well. Purse your lips and blow wind noises. Hear the sighing sounds that the wind makes. Carry on swaying and balancing as before, but now stop blowing. Instead, close your eyes and move the focus of your attention to your belly button, your navel. This is your middle, the center of the space that you occupy. Relax and observe what is happening there.

(Pause to allow the children time to feel.)

"Feel how your tummy moves in and out. Now gradually stop swaying and stand very still.

(Pause until they are all still.)

"Find your own center. Feel how it rises up from between your feet. Feel how your feet share your weight equally. How satisfying and peaceful it is to be a tall tree, breathing quietly in the forest! Enjoy this feeling for a moment. Now open your eyes slowly and tiptoe quietly to your places. We are all ready to start the lesson. Let's look at it together."

Yoga is a science

The above exercise might well be considered odd and, in the opinion of many, irrelevant to a lesson in mathematics or a foreign language. At least, that might have been the accepted view up until April 2, 1984. On this date, to many people's amazement, the Indian cosmonaut, Rakesh Sharma, took off from the Soviet base at Baikonor aboard the Soyoz T11 space capsule, with the express objective of studying the effects of yoga in weightlessness.

Over the thirty years prior to that, many people in the West had become aware through personal experience that yoga deserved to be taken seriously. However, only a small minority of these had realized that, rather than a religion, yoga was a science. The experiments of this cosmonaut, who himself was a yogi, provided remarkable support to the latter claim. We also must admit that the Russian experts regarded yoga as a means to help men adapt to living in new forms of space.

Since the Soviets were militant atheists, it was inconceivable that they would ever have allowed the discipline of yoga to be part of their research had it any link with a "religious cult". One would hardly have imagined them sending their astronauts into space in search of God!

This unlikely example shows that yoga can be considered a science with universal applications. However, what concerns us here is its relevance to education.

Whether or not our children will find themselves living in outer space and blazing new paths across the cosmos, the fact remains that they will have to learn to adapt, like the cosmonauts, to new conditions. Whatever awaits them in the 21st century, we can be sure that knowledge will increase and life become more complicated. Whether on earth or in outer space, there will be ever more information to cram into the heads of our schoolchildren!

Rather than simply overload children's brains, we should teach them resilience so that they will be able to adapt and use their creativity fully, in order to cope with change as it occurs. Yoga can prepare them right now in the classroom for the adventures that lie ahead.

Yoga in the 'class-capsule' is ready for take-off.

Walking in Yoga "sandals"

There is an old Indian story which tells of a Maharajah who set off one day with his extensive retinue on a pilgrimage to a sacred mountain. Their long and tortuous journey took them through the jungle. In those far-off days, horses and carriages did not exist and shoes had not yet been invented. Rich and poor alike, traveled barefoot. An army of servants was therefore assigned the task of placing a series of carpets before their master, so that he would not prick or bruise his feet in the spiky jungle terrain. The carpets were

5

unrolled before him, rolled up again behind him and laid out again in front of him. The convoy was magnificent, but its progress was barely perceptible.

Now it so happened that after several days traveling, while the convoy was resting, an amazing traveler could be seen, rapidly approaching the camp. He was confidently covering the rocky ground in great strides. Invited to dine with the Maharajah, he astonished the company by declaring that he would reach the sacred mountain the very next day! His host could not believe this statement and asked how he could possibly expect to arrive so quickly at their common goal.

"Look", said the stranger as he pointed to his feet. They were wrapped in animal skins. It was clear that, with his feet protected in this novel way against cuts and bruises, he could indeed overtake any caravan.

This parable has lost none of its relevance. It illustrates the difference between an arduous, complicated technology as opposed to an obvious, natural means. The wise man is he who knows how to harness effectively the resources he finds within himself in order to overcome the challenges presented to him in life. In the jungle of modern life, are we not constantly falling victim to stress, noise and pollution? Let us heed the moral of this story. We too can put on natural "sandals" of yoga, and travel easily and quickly toward our goal: success in life.

The Eight Spirals of Life: a well marked path

From time immemorial, yogis have shown people the way towards fulfillment through continuing education. Long ago an Indian sage named Patanjali mapped out the path that would enable human beings to realize their full physical and mental well-being. Patanjali's book, *Yoga Sutra*, is about "focus". In it he points out the many obstacles that arise in our effort to focus. This concise text outlines the essentials of an ancient science which has been transmitted orally from time immemorial. Today, thanks to the writing

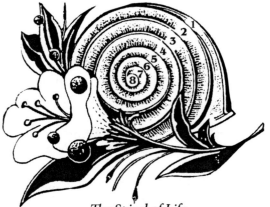

The Spiral of Life

of Patanjali, this code of universal value is available to us all.

What does he say? First and foremost, he tells us that the body and the mind are not separate entities but manifestations of the same energy, which goes from the gross to the subtle. The awakening of one's potential is carefully laid out in stages that lead slowly but surely from the external to the internal, just as the spiral of a snail's shell winds from the inside out. Grasping these life forces and gaining enhanced effectiveness in life requires patience. Let us follow the example of the independent snail which wisely carries on its back the spiral of Patanjali, the spiral of life.

In an attempt to simplify and make the Yoga Sutra understandable to all, we have summarized the essential points from the original Sanskrit text as follows: One must learn:

1. **To live together.** The path to a successful life begins with a good understanding of one's self and the environment.

2. **To drive out negative toxins and thoughts.** We become stronger by purifying our minds and bodies.

3. **To develop good posture.** We begin by learning to keep our backs upright.

4. **To breathe well so as to keep calm.** We balance our energies by acquiring proper breath control.

5. **To know how to relax in order to maintain a good energy level.** We replenish our energy through relaxation and complete the day's tasks with ease.

6. **To focus one's energy like a laser beam.** We pay better attention and remember more of what we learn.

The above stages 1 to 6 involve perfecting the intellectual faculties and sidestepping the pitfalls that are posed by the mind. They deserve our full attention, especially since our purpose is to introduce yoga to children in the classroom setting. We shall deal with them carefully in the following chapters. The next stages 7 and 8 discuss the inner life and fulfillment.

7. **To expand our consciousness.**

8. **To put ourselves on the same wavelength as the energy source.**

These last two stages deal with a private level within each and every one of us regardless of age and degree of mastery of yoga. These will not be discussed here per se, as they are not necessarily a part of day-to-day yoga practice, although elements of these stages will come to play in later parts of this book.

In teaching, we can use the body as a catalyst to learning. The stages delineated by Patanjali clearly point out the interdependence between the mind and body. It's a two way street; the mind can help to revitalize the body just as the body can help the mind perform better. We observe that sound minds give rise to balanced bodies and good health.

The yoga methods transmitted by Patanjali therefore involve gross and subtle interactions. For example, at the end of an intense mental concentration or meditation, we are taught to return to our normal conscious state gradually by means of small physical movements that make us aware of our immediate environment, smoothly and painlessly.

1

Living Together

One for all; all for one

Many people imagine yogis to be hermits with white beards living in caves in the Himalayas and spending their time meditating in a cross-legged, lotus posture. This stereotypical image is far removed from the reality of yoga which is based on relationship with oneself and with others.

Children often bring tensions to school which hamper the free flow of their energy. This translates into aggressive behavior that mimics the many violent role models they see at home and on television.

School violence increases from year to year and undermines the spirit of cooperation. At the elementary school level and sometimes even earlier, in-group fighting among pupils destroys the harmony in class, whereas experience shows that a friendly, cheerful atmosphere facilitates learning.

The child needs to become aware that he is not an isolated individual, cut off from the rest of the group. Today more than ever, children must learn to work together.

High minded concepts are one thing; applying them is something else.

Yoga is one way of incorporating what we say into what we do. It combines gestures that help us to regulate our breathing and to find our center. Yoga is an authentic life style, which integrates every cell of the body.

The exercises proposed here are designed to help children develop a sense of responsibility in relationship to their environment.

Children are lead to feel they are part of a larger group. Pupils and teachers are actively involved. The teachers are responsible for maintaining good morale among the pupils so that no child should feel left out and experience school as a failure.

EXERCISE 1 — THE MIRROR
Starting position
Students can be seated or standing.
Procedure
First Stage

- Rub your hands together vigorously until they are quite warm.
- Now bring your hands close to each other without touching them together, with palms facing each other. Feel the energy that has been generated by rubbing your hands. Now draw them away from each other little by little until you no longer feel any energy waves. Although invisible to the eye, the energy and warmth from this friction can still be felt strongly in the hands and the fingers.

Second Stage

- Pair off in partners and repeat the exercise. Energize your hands by rubbing them together and face your partner.
- Now you and your partner bring your left palms close until they are practically touching. Then gradually draw your palms apart, paying close attention to the sensation in your hand. Do the same thing now using your right hands. Repeat the exercise using both hands.

Third Stage

- Still working in pairs, decide beforehand which one of the partners would like to be the 'mirror'.

- Rub your hands together and place your left hands facing each other.
- The partner, who is going to be the 'mirror', closes his eyes. The other partner moves his hand any way he likes, but very slowly. The 'mirror' tries to follow the partner's hand movements by feeling the sensations created, but without touching or looking.

Link with Tradition

In yoga, we say that the body radiates an aura. This aura can be sensed by most people, whether they are aware of it or not, and it explains why we sometimes experience a spontaneous feeling of sympathy or of antipathy when we meet someone for the first time.

Effects

The goal of this exercise is to help develop awareness of subtle sensations which in turn allow us to develop a sense of the presence of one another. Secondly, it does away with feelings of rejection by including the children in an exercise they can all enjoy.

Best Use of this Exercise

At the start of a lesson or when there is a feeling of stress or fatigue in the classroom after the completion of an intensive study exercise.

The 'mirror' exercise is particularly effective during the first hour of class when it is cold outside and the pupils have just come indoors.

Observations

Children are quick to sense the energy emanating from the body. This exercise is valuable for students of all ages, and can be adapted to suit the teacher's lesson plan.

EXERCISE 2 —BREATHING ALL TOGETHER

Starting Position

Have the children divide up in groups of four. The pupils must remain standing throughout the duration of this exercise.

Procedure

First Stage

- You will begin by letting yourselves become aware of your own breathing, without paying attention to what your neighbor is doing. In the beginning, do not pay any attention to your neighbor. Notice the rhythm of your own breath. Begin to move your arms to the rhythm of your breathing as follows:

- *As you breathe in,* open out your arms very slowly sideways and turn them upwards, like a flower that is beginning to bloom.

- *As you breathe out,* bring your arms towards the chest and lower your head, like a flower that shuts. When you have finished exhaling, the forearms should be crossed at the front of the body.

- Be sure to synchronize the movements with your breath.

Second Stage

- Staying silent, at my signal, you will perform these movements altogether, in your group of four. All of you will move your arms outwards and inwards together at the same time. Let's start.

Third stage

- The same exercise as above, however this time the whole class does the exercise together, synchronizing their breath and the movement.

Link to Tradition

In yoga, there is a strong emphasis on the relationship between movement and breath which is the basis of what is called hatha yoga.

Effects

The rhythmic movements and synchronization of breathing induce a calming effect on each individual as well as the group.

This exercise clears the mind and sharpens thinking by increasing the flow of oxygen throughout the body, particularly to the brain.

Thanks to the simultaneous focus on oneself and on the group, interpersonal relationships are enhanced.

Best Use of this Exercise

This exercise is particularly effective when the class has been sitting for a very long time.

Observations

This exercise can be renamed in any number of ways, depending on the circumstances and needs of the class. Possible suggestions are: a flower garden or day and night.

EXERCISE 3 — THE PHARAOH'S VASE

Starting Position

If possible, have the pupils sit in a circle. The important thing is for them to be able to focus their full attention without distraction on a designated point, either in the center of the circle, or (if they are not able to sit in a circle) on something in front of them. We recommend placing a real object, such as a vase or a hat, in the center of the circle so that the children can use it as a 'receptacle' for their energy.

Procedure

- Exhaling, place the back of your hands one against the other, arms held in front of the body.

- Inhaling, extend your arms in front of you, bending the elbows and opening them upwards in the form of a vase.

- Hold your breath in and lower your arms. Cross them over in front of your chest and touch your shoulders lightly with your hands in fists.

- Breathe out while extending your arms in front of you and turning the palms upwards, all the while being aware of the movement and keeping your gaze on the chosen point.

Links with Tradition

This exercise has been handed down since the times of the pharaohs. Egyptian and Iranian statues and frescoes provide visual representations of the exercise.

Effects

This exercise helps make children aware of a potential collective energy which can be used in common creatively. Children learn to interact with each other and with the teacher who is part of the group.

This is an excellent respiratory exercise that helps open up the chest; it induces a similar openness on a psychic plane (i.e. compassion, empathy…).

Best Use of this Exercise

This exercise is best used at the beginning of the day or the week. It is especially good for rebuilding the unity within the class after a return from vacation.

A Pleasant Class

We often underestimate the powerful effects of moments such as the beginning of the school year, the commencement of a semester, the first day of a new week and the start of a new day. Everyone loves springtime and youth. Yet we do little to instill spring in the hearts of our young people. The usual school trip would perhaps have greater value at the beginning

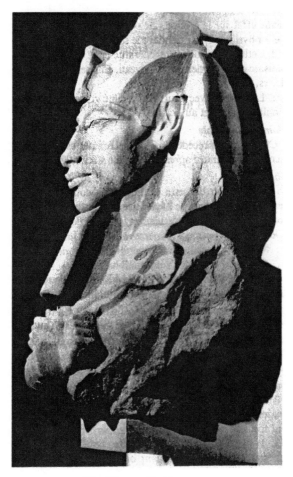

The Pharaoh's Vase

rather than at the end of the school year as a means to foster good relationships between students and their teacher from the onset. We can summarize the need in one word: *Welcome.*

In the exercises described here, we have tried to make up for this oft' forgotten "welcome". Yet we know from the most recent findings in psychology, as well as from the teachings of yore, that it is important for children to experience pleasure in being together. That pleasurable experience is a determining factor in whether we as parents and teachers succeed or fail in reaching the children in our care. We all cherish those moments when our children willingly accept a task at hand. When pupils feel a sense of belonging in the classroom or in their families, they gain confidence. We sometimes see them go on to achievements that no one would have imagined them capable of.

Whereas some looks can kill, others can give wings. This leads us to emphasize the importance of artistic expression. Yoga creates togetherness that is conducive to activities in theater, art and music.

In the scientific field, success today is no longer the result of the work of an isolated man, but of a team. The Nobel Prize, for example, is seldom awarded to a sole individual, but is shared by several scientists for a discovery which has been achieved jointly. It is imperative to prepare the young people of today to work in harmony with one another, or in other words, on the same wavelength.

2

Eliminate Toxins and Negative Thoughts

Operation Good Mood

Yoga is in complete agreement with modern psychology when it recognizes that a good sense of self is the best way to establish an atmosphere of peace and calm.

As we have seen, a positive attitude enhances confidence and puts us in step to becoming a winner. However, confidence is often undermined when we are in poor physical shape. Sometimes a grain of sand is all it takes to disrupt the entire machinery. How can we prevent this and also maintain a positive attitude in life? Yoga sets out to answer these questions.

First, yoga tells us to clean our house – the body – by eliminating body toxins. The purification process in yoga happens on a daily basis as we learn to unblock joints where negative energy has accumulated. Then, as the energy flows freely, we can cultivate a calm mind. We find that our anxieties and fears disappear and we experience a positive outlook.

And yoga assures us that the good mood which we create within ourselves will spill over into our daily environment.

Ayurvedic medicine, which is to India what acupuncture is to China, tells us that the source of many of our most common illnesses is constipation. We have all noticed that a constipated person (in every sense of the word) does not exude health and *joie de vivre*.

Few people realize that many of our modern mental health disorders could be prevented by the simple release of the blocked energies of the body. Minor modifications in our ways of eating, chewing and breathing can bring about marvelous improvements. In short, we need to become aware of the influence which our own organic functions have on our well-being. Even something as simple as a massage glove, when well applied, can do wonders for the skin! Think of it! A little bit of discipline goes a long way towards improvement.

Many people, intellectuals in particular, are sedentary and spend long hours at their desks. Why don't they develop the habit of getting up, for example, every hour, opening the window or doing some of the exercises that are written about in this chapter? Rabelais tells us the consequences this may have in the fictional portrayal of the young giant, Pantagruel, who grows lazy and stupid because his tedious teacher will not let him express his natural instincts. A minor reform in the classroom could have helped this poor little giant find balance in life.

Exercises for unblocking the joints, opening up the lungs and ventilating the brain, are part of a basic health plan for the class. It is through using the body as a springboard to better learning that the exercises taught here will be truly effective.

EXERCISE 4 — CLEANING HOUSE
Procedure

Feet (Figure ①)

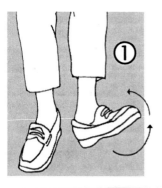

Two types of movements:

1. **Rotation:** Five times clockwise, five times anti-clockwise.

   Note: Depending on the time available, the two feet can be moved together or one after the other.

2. **Bending:** Extend the feet towards the ground and then pull them up towards the body. Repeat five times.

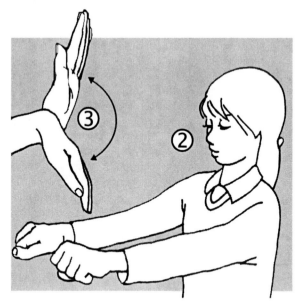

Hands

Three types of movements:

1. Alternately, open your hands out and then close them in a fist, with your thumbs on the outside: five times. (*See figure* ②.)

2. Make a fist with the thumb on the outside and rotate the wrist: five times clockwise and five times anti-clockwise.

3. Stretch out your arms in front of you: raise your palms upwards and then bend them forwards so that the fingers point to the floor: five times. (*See figure* ③.)

The teacher counts each turn out loud as the children move accordingly.

These same foot and hand exercises lend themselves well to the practice of synchronizing breath and movement. This is how to practice it:

Inhalation: On the upward movement.

Exhalation: On the downward movement.

19

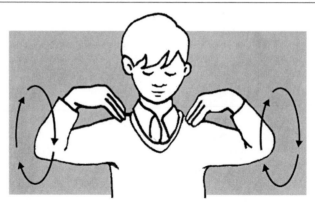

Shoulder and Arm Movements

Shoulder Rotation. Place your fingers on your shoulders; rotate the elbows (*illustration above*).

> Repeat five times backwards and five times forward. This exercise can also be done in synchronization with breathing.

Bending. Extending the forearm (*illustration below*).
To synchronize with the breath:

> Inhale slowly: Stretch out your forearms in front of you.
> Exhale slowly: Bring your forearms to the shoulders.
>
> Repeat this exercise five times.

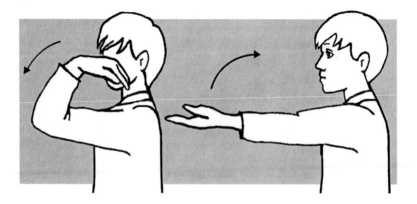

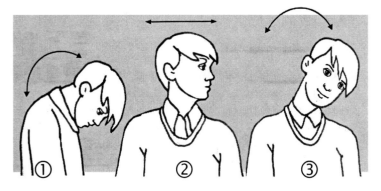

Head and Neck Rotation

① Let your head and neck fall gently forward toward the chest, and then up and backward.

② Let your head and neck fall gently sideways, first to the right shoulder, then the left.

③ Rotation: clockwise and then anti-clockwise.

Warning! These exercises must be done with caution. Be careful that the cervical vertebrae stay aligned to the dorsal axis. It is essential that the spinal column be maintained in a good upright position. Do not try to take these exercises too far forward and backward. Limit exercises ①, ②and ③ to five times in each direction.

Link with Tradition

These exercises are part one of a series of yoga exercises called *Pawanmuktasana*.

Effects

Hand and Foot Movements

These exercises are simple and require no prior training. They are part of the system of yoga for beginners. The hands and feet are important nerve centers in our body. Therefore,

21

these seemingly insignificant exercises have a balancing effect which calms as well as tones the nerves.

Shoulder and Arm movements

These promote the development of the thoracic cage and good ventilation in the lungs, which in turn, increases the flow of oxygen to the brain and improves overall muscle tone.

Head and Neck Movements

These relieve tension in the head and neck. They have calming effect, especially when synchronized with breathing. They are excellent for refocusing attention when you realize that the children are becoming restless and distracted.

Best Use of the Exercise

We recommend this series be done in the morning. However, it is also good to do it in the beginning of the afternoon after lunch, as it will not interfere with digestion. The apparent simplicity of these movements does not detract from their effectiveness in refreshing the body and mind. They are also effective exercises of dynamic relaxation, before or after writing sessions, after long periods of immobility or whenever there is a lull in concentration.

Variations

Instead of counting, you may synchronize the movements to:
> *music*
> *poetry*
> *the alphabet*
> *list of things on a particular theme.*

EXERCISE 5 — THE WOOD CUTTER
Starting Position

The students are standing.

Procedure

We will imitate a woodcutter who is cutting wood in a forest.

- Exhaling, lean slightly forward pretending to hold an imaginary axe. Place your two fists firmly one above the other.
- Inhaling deeply through the nose, raise the axe above the head. Make sure your position is correct.
- Forcefully exhaling through the mouth make the sound "HA", at the same time lowering the arms and bending the knees, as if you were splitting a huge piece of wood in two.... Go ahead, with all your strength! "HA"
- Repeat the exercise twice.

Link with Tradition

In India, this exercise is part of a series called *Shakti Bandhas*, which means these practices aim to unblock the energy flow. In addition, these purifying breathing exercises, such as the "HA" breath, are used a lot in Tibetan yoga.

Effects

The 'Wood Cutter' frees accumulated tensions in the area of the solar plexus.

It strengthens the abdominal muscles.

This exercise seems like the counter pose to sustained intellectual work, provided that one places awareness in the abdomen when exhaling and shouting "HA"

Best Use of the Exercise

When students are tense before an exam or an important event. After an extended period of mental activity.

Observations

It is very important for the "HA" sound to come from the lower abdomen and not just from the throat. In reality, the energy that enables us to cut the wood emanates from the center, the solar plexus, what the Japanese call the 'Hara'. Therefore, the "HA" sound is a natural exhalation, resulting from a sudden movement.

When confidence generates confidence

We cannot overestimate the extent to which our attitudes influence those of the children in our charge, whether in the family or at school. But to what extent do our prejudices influence the performance of our children?

Tell a teacher, for example, that some of their pupils are of above average intelligence. Let this positive prejudice simmer and then see the effect it produces: a peak in the intellectual performance by those very same pupils!

Whether you believe this or not, just such an experiment was carried out in a California school. Preliminary statistical data gave the majority of the children as coming from average backgrounds and being normal in terms of learning aptitude. In short, they were altogether, ordinary children. The purpose of the study was to show that pupils who receive more attention from their teachers will display greater progress than others. In the study, the teachers were told beforehand that some of their students were particularly gifted and that these were expected to show a spectacular intellectual development. In fact, the names of the so-called "gifted" pupils had been selected at random.

At the end of the year, it was evident beyond doubt, that the students who had been designated as being of "superior intelligence" did indeed make remarkable progress in comparison to the other children.

This experiment has since been repeated many times. Further experiments have shown that we can exercise an influence over others through our manner, without necessarily uttering a single word.

How do we produce this influence beyond words? There seems to be some unknown factor at work which we shall, for discussion purposes, label "X" and which relates to mind-to-mind communication. This X factor gives rise to one of three types of effects: positive, negative or neutral. Teachers are well aware that this X factor plays a major role in teaching, even in subjects like mathematics or chemistry.

Whether a child will succeed or fail depends in large part on the confidence his parents and teachers show in him. Our attitudes will make him love studying and want to do well in school.

A positive mental direction is absolutely necessary when we are raising children. It is without doubt the reason why so many motivated educators have found the way to yoga.

The Key Phrase that transforms you

The first step of the yogi is to realize that change for the better is possible. One method of attaining this is by means of a key phrase. This is a positive word or expression which we choose, adopt and develop for our private use and which we will try to engrave on an unconscious level through repetition. It is a powerful tool for change.

Although it is impossible to control our thoughts all the time, we can at various moments throughout the day, when the psyche is especially receptive, take time to repeat to ourselves our "key phrase". The most favorable moments are in the evening right before going to sleep, in the morning as we are waking up, before we get out of bed and at the beginning and the end of a relaxation session.

In the state between sleep and wakefulness, the whole mind is receptive and welcomes these suggestions that we give ourselves. For example, someone who is plagued with self doubt may repeat to themselves: "I have confidence in myself."

25

This key phrase will gradually take root. When the repetition is done with perseverance, the brain reorients itself in the desired direction.

Teachers and parents today are filled with second thoughts about themselves. **In our opinion, the reassessment of an educator's importance goes hand in hand with improving our system of education.**

Nothing does more harm than the constant repetition of negative thoughts. Before an exam or a test, many children are assailed with the throbbing memories of former failures. This state of mind is not conducive to collecting your strengths. On the contrary, it saps energy. Patanjali, the father of yoga, gives us a reliable trick. When the mind is overcome by fear, he advises us to evoke the opposite feeling, one that is peaceful and secure. If you are afraid of failing, recall a happy memory of success. This method is very effective and revitalizing.

Best use of the exercise

In the evening, before going to bed, make sure that you keep your thoughts positive, instead of falling into the trap of negative thinking again. As soon as you feel yourself falling asleep, repeat your key phrase three times. Do the same thing in the morning when you wake up and again, of course, during your daily relaxation session.

3

Walk Tall!

From monkey to man

Have you ever amused yourself by imitating a gorilla? If so, you have leaned forward, rounded your back and swung your arms. This act of mime immediately gives you a feel of the real animal. You can test for yourself what differentiates human beings from other primates: an erect spinal cord. The vertical position of man is the sign of his having left the animal world. All traditions insist on the straightness of the back: Tai Chi, Chiropractics, ballet, Zen and everyone's mother. Being able to sit with your back straight is an integral part of any real meditation.

Human equilibrium relies on the attraction of two poles, the earth and the sky. The Chinese say that man governs the Middle Empire. The center of gravity, situated midway between the soles of the feet and the top of the head receives particular attention by virtue of it being the center of vital energy. Within this space are joined two complementary forces, that of primitive instincts that draw us downwards and that of our aspirations that propel us upwards. Reaching towards the sky is all the more possible when the base is stable. The experience of several millennia shows that all true wisdom needs to take account of the body and of its needs before thinking of flying towards higher spheres. We are all familiar with the story about the astronomer who, by staring up so much at the stars, ended by falling down into a well. Thus, let us take care not to let the body double up and the back revert to its primeval curve. The destiny of man is not to resemble King Kong, the king of apes. All searchers agree that there exists a relationship between the straightness of the back and the development of the human brain.

The language of the body

Many of our species forget to carry themselves with a straight back, which is their distinctive feature. Consequently, their shoulders stoop, their breathing shortens and, worse than that, their self confidence diminishes significantly.

We are all familiar with the caricatures usually associated with people who have poor posture. For example, there's the intellectual with his 'head in the clouds' and his neck extended forwards who bumps into everything he comes in contact with, lost as he is in his thoughts. We also recognize the timid, shy person by his shrinking inward posture. Yet another, is the 'well built' muscle-bound athlete whose rigidity does not augur well for old age. Unless he changes his ways, he will suffer from back and knee problems later.

We call the spinal cord the 'Tree of Life'. Its straightness and daily maintenance will have a positive effect on your mind/ body/health.

Recommendation: get into the habit of adopting the position and demeanor of someone who has confidence in life. While walking, keep your back straight and breath deeply with your chest open. Keep your focus in front of you and walk with an alert step. Watch how this stance affects your inner state.

Do you have a good back?

Eighty percent of adults over the age of thirty suffer from back pain. This high percentage is due to a lack of training of the spine, which should start in school.

The lumbar area is subject to a lot of strain as a result of our upright posture. Over time, this strain gives rise to an abnormal swayback curvature of the lumbar region in the lower back that we call lordosis. It is prevalent among young people today, as well as its compensatory, hunchback curvature corollary on the level of the dorsal spinal region named, *kyphosis*. Some people go to the opposite extreme by tucking the tailbone under and pushing the pubic bone forward, leading with the hips, in an attempt to erase all primitive curvature of the back in the belief that in this way they will reach the goal of evolution more quickly. This practice seems excessive to us.

Let us restrict our practice to the following moderate exercise: **Pelvic "See-Saw"** to relieve the lumbar region. It is an essential exercise before practicing any backward stretches. If there is room to stretch out, lie down on your back, feet on the floor, legs bent at a 90° angle. Become aware of the lumbar curve. At this level, you will probably feel a small bridge. Slip your hand under the arch of your back. Contract the muscles of the abdomen and let your back press down on your hand. Then remove your hand and feel the back fully flat on the ground, the arch being obliterated, which – while not being the correct alignment - gives you the sensation of one extreme. Then move your pelvis in the opposite direction, arching the lumbar and pushing your butt into the floor.

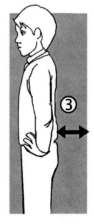

Repeat this see-saw movement several times. This exercise can also be performed from a seated or a standing position. If done standing, it is best to flex the knees slightly, stomach tucked in and buttocks lightly clenched. It is recommended to place the hands at the pelvis, to feel the movement of the see-saw better. *(Picture ③)*.

Opening up the chest to straighten the dorsal region : the curved back almost always accompanies a wide gap between the shoulder blades. The entire scapular area should be exercised. The exercises of 'candelabra' *(page 35)* and 'shoulder and arm movements' *(page 20)*

Standing position for Pelvic See-Saw

are excellent for reconditioning the dorsal vertebrae.

Arrange the cervical vertebrae on the spinal axis by making a double chin, looking directly in front of you. The shoulders remain low and pressed down.

No more hunched backs

The standing, upright position is the most commonly held from the time human beings learn to walk. However, few people know how to stand correctly, for the simple reason that correct posture is not taught in schools. Yoga attaches great importance to posture. The first task of the teacher is to teach correct sitting and standing positions.

How well we function intellectually depends in large part on how well we sit. We listen best when our back is straight, in a manner of speaking, when our antenna is properly aligned.

EXERCISE 6 — THE CORRECT STANDING POSTURE

Procedure

- **Feel the contact with the ground**. Distribute the body weight equally between both feet.

- **Knees.** Turn the kneecaps slightly outwards by rotating the inner thigh forward.

- **Pelvic basin.**

- **Upper back**. Bring together the shoulder blades, lowering the shoulders, relaxing them, towards the back.

- **Nape of the neck.** Slightly lower the chin so that the nape of the neck is straight but not rigid.

- **Relax the face.**

Now you are ready to deal with all the standing postures.

Link with Tradition

Tadasana, a posture where you stretch upwards.

Effects

Physical. Corrects the defects of the back
Mental. This posture increases confidence in oneself.

Yoga of the Forest

The famous yogi Goraknath, often said to be the "father" of Hatha Yoga, catalogued the 84,000 postures – called *asanas*. This legendary sage brought together a team of 'zoologists' from the 'best university' so to speak, the forest, and he collected their keen observations of nature. The result of these observations produced the repertory of well known postures, a number of which have been named after animals, such as the cobra (*bhujangasana*), the locust (*shalabhasana*), and the eagle (*garudasana*). The original Sanskrit names deserve to be kept by the teachers of yoga so as to preserve the link with time-honored wisdom.

These graphic postures can be greatly enjoyed in school and have wide appeal among pupils. Children are very close to the mineral, plant and animal worlds. These postures coded by Tradition offer the advantage of channeling their primitive energies. Moreover, they have a beneficial impact on the endocrine glands. They are especially recommended for teenagers as they confront the biological storm of puberty.

How to present these postures to children

Make note of these key points:

1. **Children enjoy movement.** Whereas long periods of sitting is familiar to adults, it is generally counter-indicated for children. Sustained sedentary work puts pressure on the fragile ligaments and cartilage of the young body and is not suitable for a child's spine, which is still very malleable.

For this reason, the posture sequences presented here are rapid and attractive.

2. **Teach children not to punish their bodies.** The competitive tendency must be controlled and should never lead children to show off and act against natural movement. Pain is the 'red light' which should make children moderate their practice.

3. **Teach them to be aware of their bodies by being conscious of their movements.** Raising the arms attentively, while synchronizing breath and movement, is much better than forcing a difficult pose on the children with the intention of dazzling an audience. Any act performed mindfully is worth its weight in gold.

EXERCISE 7 — A SHORT SALUTATION TO WORK

Starting position

Have the children push their chairs back slightly, asking them to be very careful to lift the chairs quietly in order to prevent making noise. Their chests need to be around 20 centimeters away from the edge of the desk.

Procedure

- Remaining seated, straighten the back and sit in an upright position. Relax the neck, drop the shoulders and bring your chin down to the chest. Relax the back. Relax the whole body and breathe in and out calmly, keeping the body absolutely still *(See figure ①.)*

- *Inhaling*, raise your arms in front of you, paying attention so that you do not bend. Once you have inhaled fully,

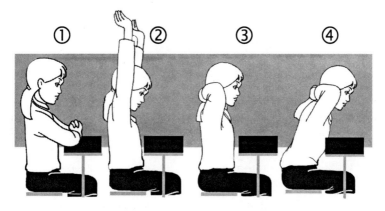

the arms should be stretched above the head and slightly towards the back. (*See figure* ②.)

- *Exhaling,* bend the forearms. Make a tight fist with each hand and press them together at the back of the neck. This should exert a strong pressure on the head, as if you wanted to press it forward; however the head must resist and stay in place. These two opposing forces cancel out each other but they result in an increased firmness and the straightness of the spinal column. (*See figure* ③.)

- *Inhaling,* remain straight and firm. Prepare yourself to maintain this position for the duration of the exercise, with the elbows spread out towards the back,

- *Exhaling,* lean forwards like a plank being lowered. The back stays perfectly straight and the movement stops once your chest touches the desk. (*See figure* ④.)

  Attention! The nape of the neck should not bend. To help the head maintain the correct position, fix your gaze on a point straight in front of you.

- *Inhaling,* slowly raise the chest, your back completely straight and your head firmly held. Return to the upright position. (*See figure* ③.)

- *Exhaling,* slowly lower the arms and bring them to the side of the body.

This is the end of the exercise. Relax your body. Feel the back toned; it remains upright on its own, without too much effort!

Link with Tradition

This exercise is inspired by *Surya Namaskar*, the "Sun Salutation" that all students of yoga are well acquainted with.

Effects

We have noticed that children are unable to sit up straight when they are told to do so. They need exercises that make them aware of their backs and enhance muscle tone. The spinal column can be compared to the mast of a ship, another strong image that impacts children's imaginations. A mast has strong ropes that help it to remain straight. Many muscles and ligaments perform this role. Their job is to maintain the vertebrae in place and to prevent their compression. If we want their continued service throughout our lifetime, it is imperative to train them properly by regular exercise. The short salutation at work was conceived with this goal in mind.

Additionally, the movements should be synchronized with breathing. In this way, they will automatically be performed slowly. The practice can have a very profound impact on the deeper muscular layers, which in turn stimulate the various body organs.

Best Use of this Exercise

When students have been seated writing for a long period. Do not practice after meals.

Observations

The exercise is rather difficult to perform. You should not expect success the first time round. Many students want to place their chest over the table, without realizing that what they are doing is ineffective if they let their heads fall or the back curl.

The teachers will accept the imperfect beginning. Their

patience will be rewarded. The effect is worth the wait. The children will realize that they will be able to straighten their backs. Usually, they will start out by finding this exercise difficult and then – surprise, surprise – they will start asking for it over and over again – as if they understand that, when they have not done it for a while, their backs become lazy. They learn the result is worth the effort.

EXERCISE 8 — CANDELABRA

Starting Position

Students stand in an upright position, arms at the side of the body as in exercise 6. They position themselves in such a way as to have enough space.

Procedure

- **Exhale** fully.
- **Inhale** and flex your forearms and bring your hands to the shoulders, elbows against the body. *(See figure ①.)*
- **Exhale** in the same position.

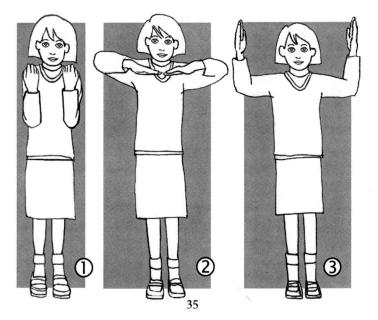

35

- **Inhale** and raise the elbows sideways, arms parallel to the ground. *(See figure ②.)*
- **Exhale** in the same position.
- **Inhale** and raise the forearms at right angles to the upper arms. Tuck in the chin and bring the shoulder blades together, drawing the elbows backwards. *(See figure ③.)*
- **Exhale** in the same position.
- **Inhale** and maintain the position of the arms in candelabra.
- **Exhale** and lower the hands on the shoulders and
- **Inhale** in this position.
- **Exhale** and bring the elbows to the sides of the body and
- **Inhale** in this position.
- **Exhale** and lower the forearms.

(End of the exercise)

Link with Tradition

This is a popular exercise in Irano-Egyptian yoga.

Effects

This exercise tones the whole back, above all the dorsal region, which is badly affected in the classroom setting.

This exercise expands the chest and thereby increases the volume of oxygen inhaled.

The candelabra posture is known to favor the development of self-confidence and an attitude of openness towards others.

Observations

This exercise is more complicated for children than it seems when it comes to placing their hands in the candelabra position. It can be done in pairs, one pupil correcting the other.

The candelabra exercise is recommended when studying ancient Egypt in history classes. Pupils will appreciate the importance attached by the early Egyptians to the proper maintenance of the body.

4

Breath is Life

Find time to breathe

Nothing better reveals the relation between breathing and the mind than the voice of good common sense. Let us listen to what it has to say:

> *Take time to breathe.*
> *You are out of breath.*
> *Do not model yourself on people of shallow breath.*

If your loving grandmother saw you running about endlessly, she would have the wind knocked out of her and she would plead with you to catch your breath.

Why be in such a big hurry to get to your final breath? Make the decision now to take a breather; set aside a little time in the course of each day for yoga. While doing so, you will hear your loved ones heave a sigh of relief.

Age-old Advice

From ancient times, breath has been associated with a vital energy. The word *prana* used in yoga corresponds to:

> *Chi* in Chinese
> *Ki* in Japanese
> *Rouah* in Hebrew
> *Pneuma* in Greek
> *Anima* in Latin
> *Baraka* in Arabic

Prana is part of the cosmos. It knows no frontiers, requires no passport. It travels with breath but it is not breath. It is as imperceptible to us as the nucleus of an atom.

Our lungs put us in contact with the very subtle energies which provide nourishment to our blood and being. Are we not told that God breathed life into Adam's nostrils and set him thus on his exceptional destiny? Incidentally, mankind has not always measured up to the expectations of that divine start.

Prana is not confined to breath alone. It is also present in the flavor of food and the pleasure given by a fine sight, a fragrant perfume or a beautiful piece of music. It can be found in an exchange of kind words. But above all, it gives manifold strength to those who know how to keep their thoughts and minds focused on the positive aspects of life.

Breathing in Yoga—a way to re-energize

Article No. 1 of your personal Constitution should be to breathe correctly. Governed by the autonomous nervous system, breath can be presided over by your willful intervention via the central nervous system, that is to say – Mister Brain.

It is possible to sense this when we breathe with our whole body and not only with our lungs. When you feel the sensation of breathing in each fiber of your body, you will experience a sense of profound well-being. Awareness of this deep full breathing unlocks the potential for mastery over our body organs, and therefore is an important factor in maintaining good health.

EXERCISE 9 — CONSCIOUS BREATHING
Procedure

- Keeping your back straight, sit up comfortably. With your mouth closed, begin to become aware of your nostrils. Focus all your attention on this small area, observing first the passage of air. 'I know that I am breathing in; I know that I am breathing out.' At this point, do not try to modify the duration of your breath. You are not a bellows.

- Try to breathe as if you were smelling a very delicate perfume, as if you wished to avoid awakening someone sleeping very close to you. Breathe in and out very gently and observe this quietly. You will notice that your breathing is uneven. Do you notice that one nostril is more open than the other? After practicing this for five minutes, check to see whether you are breathing more evenly or whether your breathing has spontaneously slowed down.

Link with Tradition

This exercise is the starting point of *pranayama*, the science of breathing. Buddhist yoga calls it *anapana* and it serves as the basic technique for the meditation practice of *vipassana*, single pointed focus.

Effects

To observe your breathing, you have to be focused. This life-sustaining function of the body is normally done at an unconscious level. When you become aware of this process on a daily basis, you will derive great benefits from it in your daily life.

Breathing at all levels—a test

Set aside this book for a moment and close your eyes. As you continue breathing, observe your body closely. Identify where you feel your breath. (Pause). Now open your eyes, and mark down where you experienced breath most, in your :

Abdomen?

Chest?

Nostrils and throat?

Interpretation of Test Results
*(note: The following results apply to this exercise only and present
no significant psychological value outside this context.)*

- If you marked number 3, you were involved in an intellectual activity, which was hardly surprising since prior to that you had been wholly engrossed in the reading.

- If you marked number 2, your preoccupation at that moment was of an affective nature and perhaps the required observation had aroused some kind of emotional reactions.

- If you felt your breath in number 1, the abdominal region: you kept your feet on the ground, unless a primal instinct, like hunger, was torturing you at that moment.

These three stages of respiration correspond to the three levels of our being that range from instinct to intellect:

Low Breath. The abdominal zone corresponds both with our primal instinctive impulses and our sense of being anchored in concrete reality. This is the base of our individual nature.

Middle Breath. The thoracic region is linked with our affective/emotional reactions. When we are enthused about something, we "take it to heart" and there is no way of telling where our aroused emotions will lead us.

High Breath. This zone, from the collarbone or clavicle, is linked with our mental function. It can be as much the sign of a state of mental concentration as one of mental agitation— has everything gone to your head? If so, take time to move your focus down towards the abdominal region. Feel the gentle movement at the level of your navel. Place your fingers just above the navel and get a good sense of this pulse of life.

We have often carried out this test in the classroom to check the accuracy of these interpretations. For example, after a football match, students spontaneously would focus their attention on the abdomen. Before a tough written exam or when they dread the consequences of being late, they had a natural tendency to experience their breath in the chest region. Moreover, many remarked a "racing heart". Lastly, in the course of a lesson that required intense concentration, students noticed that they had a shortened breath.

Perfect breathing does not lie in the predominance of one type of breathing over the others but in the harmony of their combined actions.

A full complete respiration is one of the important conquests of yoga.

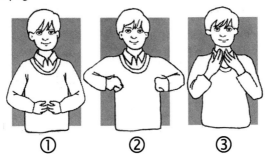

① ② ③

EXERCISE 10 — COMPLETE RESPIRATION

Preparation for the exercise —Feeling breath at three levels

Students can be seated or be standing.
They will explore their breath using their hands.

Abdominal and Diaphragmatic Breathing (*figure* ①): place one hand on the navel and the other a little bit higher. Breathe out through the nose and feel a hollow under your palms. Breathe in, and in contrast, feel your palms being pushed upwards. This constitutes one breath. Repeat this exercise several times.

Thoracic Breathing (*figure* ②): the hands, fingers curled in, are placed in the hollow of the armpits. Breathing in, feel your sides move in and out like an accordion.

Clavicular Breathing (*figure* ③): the hands are placed in the hollow of the collar bones, fingers extended towards the top of the chest. Feel this upper area move up and down with each breath.

Procedure—A growing tree

- **Exhale** (*figure* ①) and incline your head towards the front and bend your chest forwards. (*figure* ②) Place the hands back to back and bring them on a level with your legs. Do not use force! (*figure* ③)

- **Inhale** and come up taking care that the knees remain slightly bent and place your hands on them. At the end of the movement, the forearms should be in front of the chest and next to each other. Cup the hands together with palms facing forward. (*figure* ④)

- **Exhale** in this position.

- **Inhale** and extend your elbows out to your sides as far as possible so that they are level with your shoulder blades. (*figure* ⑤) Unfold the forearms on either side of you.

- **Exhale** in this position.

- **Inhale** gently and extend both arms vertically above the head. Make sure the back stays upright. (*figure* ⑥)

- **Exhale** and form the picture of a tree. (*figure* ⑦) Lower your arms to your sides in a slow and continuous movement. (*figure* ⑧) Once you have exhaled completely the arms should once again be alongside of your body. (*figure* ⑨)

  Repeat this exercise two to three times and observe what you feel.

Link with Tradition

For yogis, this exercise is the ABC of *pranayama*, the science of breathing. This practice results in a complete respiratory cycle, performed with full awareness.

Effects

These breathing techniques represent a real education in health. They have a preventive effect by reducing the chances of infection in the respiratory system.

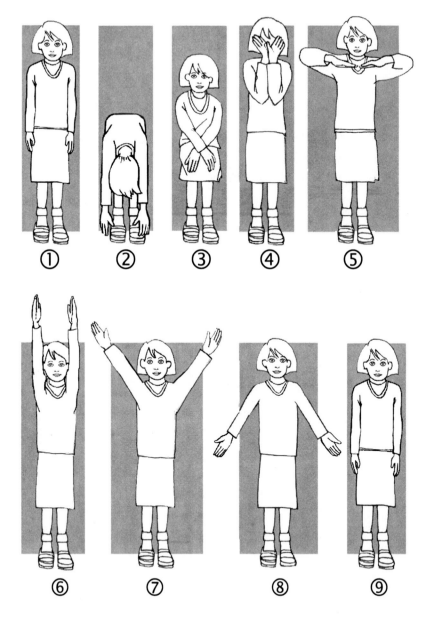

The complete breath allows a better oxygenation of the brain and thereby improves awareness and memory.

In more general terms, this exercise is one of the best remedies against phobia and anxiety. Our breathing, when complete, undoes the harmful effects of destructive emotions. The advantages are too many to be listed exhaustively. This technique is a basis of good physical and mental hygiene.

Best Use of this Exercise

Before a test or exam.
Whenever the body is gripped with tension.

Observations

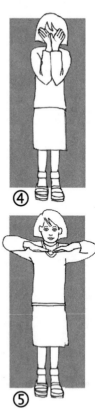

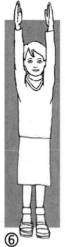

It is obvious that *a growing tree* exercise allows for complete respiration:
• When the forearms are in front of the chest (*figure* ④) you take a **low** breath; air naturally enters the abdomen while the arms and the elbows prevent it from spreading further.

• When you raise your elbows to the sides (*figure* ⑤) and you unfold the forearms, you perform a **middle** breath; the sides, drawn out by the movement of the arms, stretch to their maximum.

• Finally, the raising of the arms above the head creates a **high** breath. (*figure* ⑥)

There are many ways to perform the growing tree; instead of exhaling each time in the position, you can open up the branches in one single inhalation, which is actually more difficult.

A breath that harmonized the right side with the left

Our life depends on the healthy circulation of energy. It functions in the same manner as a bulb that you light up and the battery that you put into your tape recorder, i.e. to work properly it requires two poles: a (+) pole and a (–) pole. According to yogis, this polarization can be found throughout the body and especially at the level of the nostrils, the left being (–) and the right being (+). The interplay of these two poles, is our life-sustaining balance.

Medical science is well aware of this alternating level of the nervous system. A neurological dysfunction creates all kinds of trouble for the body. For example, if the parasympathetic system dominates, the child is lethargic. If, on the contrary, the sympathetic system is hyperactive, the child will be agitated, as is frequently the case today among young people. The acceleration of these vital functions disrupts sleep.

Yoga offers a simple method to re-balance the nervous system by means of polarized breathing exercises. These have been proven effective over and again by:

1. their calming action on students who are excited and
2. their stimulating action on students who are lethargic.

45

EXERCISE 11 — ALTERNATE BREATHING THE TRIANGLE

Starting Position: seated still with straight back, eyes open.

Procedure

First Stage

- The teacher draws an **isosceles triangle** on the blackboard and says to the class:

"Look at the angle at the bottom left. Breathe in and go up along the left side until you reach the top. The eyes should follow the movement exactly *(pause)*. Breathe out and descend along the right side *(pause)*. Breathe in and again go up along the right side *(pause)*. Breathe out and descend along the left side *(pause)*. This constitutes one round of the triangle. Repeat this exercise for a few more rounds breathing along the sides of the triangle. *(Long pause)*. Now, breathe three more times, letting your gaze follow both sides of the triangle at once."

A cycle of alternate breathing

Arrow 1: breathe in
Arrow 2: breathe out
Arrow 3: breathe in
Arrow 4: breathe out

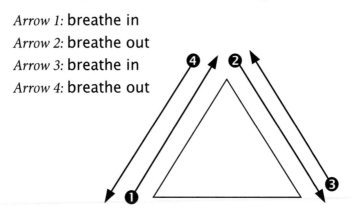

Second Stage

- The teacher continues, saying:

"Close your eyes and try to see the triangle internally, as if the two sides of the triangle coincide with your nostrils, and imagine that the summit is situated at the eyebrow center *(pause)*. Make the sides of the triangle sparkle *(pause)*. Continue breathing in the same manner while following the breath through the nostrils: breathe in from the left; breathe out from the right; breathe in from the right; breathe out from the left *(long pause)*. Now, breathe in three times from both nostrils together, along the length of the two sides of the triangle.

Third Stage

- After some months, once the students are able to perform the alternate breathing through the two nostrils with ease, the teacher can introduce a pause of two seconds between inhalation and exhalation, at the summit of the triangle between the eyebrows.

Link with Tradition

Anuloma viloma, mental alternate breathing

Effects

- This exercise harmonizes neurological functions. It develops concentration.
- It automatically induces concentration on a point at the eyebrow center which has a toning effect on the pineal gland, a very important focus during puberty.

Best Use of this Exercise

The practice of this basic exercise can begin at any time in life, from the primary school level, to middle and high school and, with variations, all the way to university... throughout adulthood!

Observations

We usually ask adult practitioners in this exercise to use their fingers to close the nostrils. With practice, we will sometimes ask older students to do the same. The principal reason we do not insist too much with young children is because they often have blocked nostrils. Also, the alternate movement of the fingers may take their attention away from the main focus of the exercise, breathing.

The advice of yogis: "breathe through the nose"

Almost all yogic breathing is through the nose and not the mouth. Certain techniques of western psychology, like bio-energy or rebirth require breathing through the mouth with a rapid rhythm. This process is useful but with the help of a psychotherapist when one wants to be freed from suppressed negative emotions. Yoga uses oral respiration in very moderate doses, for example, at the start of a course when it is necessary to clear the lungs through a sonorous 'HA' sound, typical of Tibetan yoga.

As a general rule, we recommend that students be taught to breathe through the nose. This, for two reasons:

1. It is well known that the nasal cavity tempers and purifies the surrounding air before it enters the trachea and the bronchial tubes. We all know how blocked noses mean oral breathing that increases the risk of chronic sinus and bronchial infection.

2. Breathing through the nose massages the brain via the sinuses, which act as moderators. According to yogis, there is a link between the awakening of intelligence and the passage of breath through the nose. We have all observed that one of the most striking characteristics among mentally retarded children, is that they breathe in through an open mouth.

Recommendation

If one of your students complains that he cannot breathe with his mouth closed and this state continues from one semester to the next, inform the parents and ask them to have their child examined by a medical doctor.

In conclusion, let us repeat that correct breathing is essential for our well-being. Furthermore, being aware of the flow of breath in the nostrils stimulates the brain and makes us worthy to be called *Homo sapiens*.

If we were to choose among all the practices of yoga, that one which was the most beneficial for humanity today, we would reply without hesitation: Conscious Breathing. Imagine for once what would happen if all the inhabitants of a country were to practice correct breathing for a quarter of an hour daily!

Try it out for yourself. Find that quarter of an hour daily! Practice these breathing techniques three times a day: five minutes in the morning, five minutes in the afternoon, and five minutes in the evening.

5

Stay alert and keep fit through relaxation

Rest, a law of life

Just as photos are developed in a darkroom, information gets imprinted in our brains thanks to rest. Today, due to technological progress, we know that radioisotopes enable us to observe the variations in blood circulation within the brain. A given mental activity is characterized by a surge of blood in a particular zone of the brain. These modifications are represented as images projected on a screen by means of a computer.

One of these figures shows us visually the importance of pauses in teaching: 'It has been noted that a subject who is resting and does not see anything, does not hear anything and does not move, still has an entire part of the brain, the frontal lobes, active and working. This proves that once we have stopped speaking and presenting information to students, the part of their brain that deals with processing the information continues to function long afterwards. If we introduce pauses in our lessons, we will allow for students time to process the lesson. It is necessary to teach young people to interweave periods of rest in their working time so that they disconnect and process the information. These recent scientific discoveries prove what great educators have always known, namely, that relaxation is not a diversion or an invitation to be idle but a learning tool. It has been proven that a text is memorized better if you read it before falling asleep. It seems that our brain works during the night to facilitate the absorption of knowledge. We can notice the difference the next day.

Short breaks for relaxation, interspersed into class planning in various forms, are the very pauses the brain needs to direct and assimilate information received. There is a time for everything.

Imitate a tortoise

We need to channel the often irrepressible energy of children who want to see, touch, listen to and question everything all at once. For them it is a matter of absolute necessity. Young beings, who have been confined to the womb for nine months, have to extend their antennae outwards to explore the world better and attain their full potential. Let us respect and encourage this zest for discovery in children by educating their senses.

It is well known how American Indians taught their children to recognize the gallop of buffaloes even when they were still miles away, simply by putting their ears to the ground. This ability was developed to the point where they could determine how far away the herd was and estimate its size.

But should we be perpetually on alert, so to speak, for the sake of our yoga practice? Of course not! Our senses also need a rest. For example, the eyes can rest while the ears are hard at work. Very often we will close our eyes to be able to listen more carefully. By resting, we mean shutting down our outer senses so that we can connect with our inner ones.

The thousand-year-old tradition of yoga gives us a picturesque image of relaxation by comparing it to the behavior of a tortoise that retracts all its limbs and its head into its shell.

Young people today are exhausted by the multitude of audiovisual gadgets; like adults, they spontaneously experience the need to protect themselves from the messages that assail them from all sides.

There is a time for seeing the things that surround you, and a time when you contemplate images that emerge from within. There is a time when you hear the surrounding noises, and a time when you hear the soft flutter of your breath, so close, so intimate that you might have forgotten it until then. You find yourself, as they say so well in ancient Zen texts, 'returning to the house'.

Some time ago, people discovered the pleasure of isolation boxes invented by Professor John Lily. Through simple, gentle means, we can help children break free from their external distraction and focus on subtler sensations that are taking place within their bodies. This break with the old regime enables them to recover their dissipated energies and to redirect them. They will begin their lessons on a good footing, which is precisely the objective of the exercises that follow.

EXERCISE 12—SHORT SALUTATION TO REST

Starting Position

The students, who have just spent many hours working, are seated. The teacher asks them to put down their pens and pencils, and says:

"You have worked hard. Now let's rest for a little while. Open your book to page... . After we've rested for a while, you will read this text in silence."

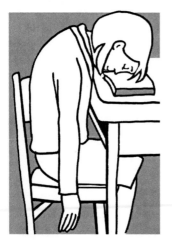

Procedure

The teacher continues saying,

"As you breathe out, lower your head and let your back slump forward. Slowly place your forehead on the table and let your arms hang loosely on both sides of the chair. Make yourself completely comfortable in this position, so that you will not feel the need to move at all for the next few minutes.

Let your awareness wander to the parts of the body that I will name and mentally repeat them after me: the soles of your feet, the legs, the buttocks on the chair, your back, right arm, left arm, both arms together, the back of the head, your forehead against the table, your nose; the tongue in your mouth, your teeth, palate, throat, head and neck, chest, abdomen, the whole body, the whole body, the whole body. Feel the body becoming very heavy.

Now, move your fingers *(pause)*. Move the toes in your shoes *(pause)*. Breathing in, raise yourself, very slowly *(pause)*. Open your eyes, focus on a color that is near you and just watch it in silence *(pause)*. Now let's begin the work that we discussed before the relaxation."

Link with Tradition

This exercise is an adaptation of the famous posture of *yoga mudra,* in the sitting position.

Effects

This position allows for the lowering of the head which in turn facilitates:
- the irrigation of the brain and
- the slowing down of sensory activity.

The brain relaxes and is refreshed. The heart beat slows down.

Bringing to mind each part of the body brings the children back to physical awareness and provides a good transitional change.

Best use of the Exercise

This exercise is particularly effective when we are mentally and/or physically exhausted.

Observations

There are many variations to this exercise. For example, the students can also place their heads on their arms on the table.

This short salutation to rest is the counter pose of the short salutation to work *(exercise 7, chapter 3)*. But they needn't be performed together.

It is important to have the students engaged immediately in a simple activity as soon as they finish the relaxation. This allows the energies, which have been recuperated, to be channelled properly.

EXERCISE 13 — THE LULLABY

Starting Position

The students are seated on their chairs and their books are open to the page of the lesson being taught.

Procedure

- "Relax your body and close your eyes *(pause)*. Listen to the surrounding sounds *(pause)*. Now, focus your attention on the sound of your breath; it is a very soft sound; pay close attention." *(pause)*

- "I will tell you what you need to do. Listen carefully and then follow the instructions. In a moment, you will block your ears with your index fingers, keeping your head and back upright. You will be able to hear the sound of your breath inside your body very clearly. Then, keeping your mouth closed, you will exhale like this – the teacher should make the audible sound 'mmmmm'. You will repeat this exercise five times. Remember to keep count correctly. And now, over to you!"

  The students perform the exercise (long pause).

- "Remove your fingers from your ears. Open your eyes. Listen now as I re-read today's lesson."

Link with Tradition

This is a variation of the *Bhramari,* which means 'bumble bee' in Sanskrit.

Effects

This exercise is both a breathing exercise and a relaxation technique that prepares us for the sensory withdrawal that we spoke of earlier.

Lengthening exhalation always has a calming effect, which is amplified when the mouth is closed and the exhalation is vibrated. This sonorous emission helps release tension while counting the cycles enhances awareness.

Best Use of the Exercise

This exercise is excellent after an intense intellectual exercise. It can also be used when students are over excited after a recreational activity.

Observations

In most languages we find the sound 'mmmmm' as the beginning sound for the word 'mother'. This shows the intimate connection between our psyche and this primordial sound.

The method of blocking the ears: traditionally, we place the index fingers inside the auditory canal, with the palms open and facing front like the surface of a radar disc.

For greater convenience, you can at first adopt an easier position: with palms on the cheek, we apply pressure on the tragus with the index fingers flat.

While making the sound 'mmmm', you can visualize the color blue, which is associated with a calming effect. Children greatly enjoy working with colors.

EXERCISE 14 — CLOSING THE DOORS

Starting Position

Sit up with straight back.

Procedure

The teacher addresses the students:

- "I want you to look at me and listen carefully. Do not follow me for the moment. I am first going to demonstrate an exercise called 'closing the doors'. Imagine that your head is a house, and your eyes and your ears are the doors. To rest the eyes, close your eyelids and gently place your index fingers on the line of the eyelashes. I will shut my ears with the thumbs. Now I can hear nothing. To relax my tongue, I roll it back lightly against the palate, mouth closed."

The teacher demonstrates as she explains the exercise.

- "When you close all the doors, you can hear your breath very well, like the waves rolling on the sand. You will count seven waves. Then, very slowly, you will remove your hands and open your eyes."

- The students perform the exercise.

Link with Tradition

This exercise is a simplified version of the technique of *shanmukhi mudra,* that means "closing the seven gates."

Effects

Closing the doors is a powerful practice that students relate to immediately. It allows them to rest the senses and to withdraw for awhile from the external world.

Best use of the Exercise

We recommend this practice when students are worn out by continual outside noise, especially towards the end of the day. This is truly a rejuvenating experience for the mind.

Suggestions

As outlined in the previous exercises, it is good to have a preset exercise for students to work on silently as soon as they have opened their eyes.

Ensure that the transition is very smooth in order to avoid the shock of contrast between internal and external perceptions.

6

Gather together your forces, like a Laser Ray

The mind—a racing computer

Educating is a difficult task in today's world. We cannot single-handedly come to grips with boredom, disenchantment, drug use and rampant violence and bring them to the ground. These evils of society are beyond our means of intervention. Therefore, we will not waste our time on them but will spend it more usefully by focusing on another modern day plague that threatens the future of the rising generation: the distracted mind.

This problem is the root cause of many of our society's ills, referred to earlier.

It seems as if the excessive stimulation caused by our way of life has the initial effect of overexciting the mind. Much like a racing car engine, it roars in panic. We have often seen the allegory in science fiction where the robot suddenly goes berserk. The confused circuits create a disturbing cascading effect, all the more harmful as a long, suspenseful time lapses before those persons in charge manage to find the lever capable of stopping this havoc!

If we take a close look at this, we realize that the failure of our children in school is in direct relationship with our inability as educators to understand the type of mind that promotes a well-balanced individual. Our shortcoming in this area has incalculable consequences on the economy of a country and is one of the major contributing factors of the rampant crisis in our schools.

From the large volume of mail which we receive containing questions about the methods developed by RYE over the course of the last decades, there is one recurring theme : the unanimous request by teachers that we provide them with means for recovering and developing children's ability to pay attention.

Any easy explanation begs the question, "how can we expect children to learn when they cannot even listen?" What chance do they have of being good students if they cannot focus their attention?

This is exactly the domain in which yoga is King. Yoga teaches us about and shows us how to concentrate.

The eye of a bird

A story from Vedic literature offers us a good visual example of concentration. Drona, a character from the famous epic tale, *Mahabharata*, is tutoring the five Pandava brothers in the art of archery. One day he takes them into the forest and asks one of them to draw his bow and aim it towards a tree.

"What can you see?" asks Drona.

"I can see a bird on a branch," replies the boy.

"That is not enough," says Drona and he turns to the next Prince. "And about you, Arjuna, what can you see?"

"I see the eye of the bird perched on the branch."

"Good, you know the art of archery," says Drona.

Concentration is not possible unless we unify the divergent tendencies of the mind in order to achieve a precise goal and only one. The goal is to gather the scattered beams of attention, that are usually dispersed through the various areas of the senses, and to focus them on a central point which becomes the target. Today, one of the more spectacular of scientific inventions, remarkable because of its efficacy in a variety of domains, allows us to understand concentration better: the laser beam. A luminous and concentrated jet, it is able to exert an exceptionally powerful effect and to pierce the most opaque walls. A person who is expert at concentration can operate similarly.

Record knowledge... in high fidelity

The teacher must realize that there exists, consciously or unconsciously, a certain latency between the registration and the recitation of the lesson. It is not enough to read, hear and transcribe a text. Before asserting that it is learned, it is necessary to process information internally, to create a sort of "mind management" in much the same way as a computer functions.

Teachers must be well versed in the techniques of internal acquisition of knowledge so that they can teach children how to learn optimally. As mentioned previously, calming the mind is the first stage. The second stage consists in remaining aware so that we can evoke internally, at will, the sensations and concepts we have received. Just as in a Hi-Fi stereo, the quality of the recording determines the quality of the reproduction.

Up until very recently, educational science has not been very concerned with this phenomenon. Today, research findings such as those of Antoine de la Garanderie confirm the ancient wisdom of *Raja Yoga*. He has shown that when an educator succeeds in focusing the dissipated mind of a child, teaching becomes an easy task.

Can a cracked mirror reflect a landscape? One must first repair the mirror.

Today, the child's mind is overtaxed due to family, society and endocrine factors. We definitely need to look for corrective measures to these various disorders through suitable means, but we cannot afford the luxury of waiting for the family, society and medicine to fix things in due course. We need to act now as teachers, using simple methods, and give children the means to help themselves. Here is what the teacher can and must do: create in the student a state of awareness.

How do we get there?

Two methods for creating a state of awareness:

1. Ask the child to focus on a point. While this is a simple task for those learners at the top of the class, the average student will find it to be easier said than done.

2. Ask the students to shut their eyes and to use '*dharana*'. This Sanskrit word that we translate loosely as recovered concentration, is a complex but essential process which can best be defined as the mental evocation of a sensory impression.

For example, I can recreate within me an image or recall a sound or phrase that I have seen in the external world. I should also be able to imagine a certain smell, the taste of the chocolate I have just eaten, to feel the tactile sensation of velvet or the bark of a tree. Through this experience, we can train children to reproduce internally the stimuli that they have experienced. In this manner, knowledge that we are conveying will not remain tasteless and dry but will become concrete and alive. Students will not only be able to reproduce the information better but also, because of the subtle sensory experiences, be able to use it and invent new concepts.

Creativity will benefit immensely through the intensive cultivation of the inner senses.

All ears or all eyes—
Everyone has his own way of remembering

We will notice that all students do not have the same sensory capacity. This becomes the decisive factor which allows us to discover the form of teaching most appropriate to each one. For example, for some, the auditory system is more sensitive while for others, it is the visual system. We will still find other students whose motor skills are especially well developed.

These observations should not in any event be used to categorize students for life. Nothing is more harmful to the development of a young person than a premature classification that carries with it the risk of being false, thereby closing the door to his dormant potentials. If a child is an auditory learner, he must not stick to this style alone but seek to develop the other senses as well in order to avoid an imbalance.

This is one of the multiple reasons to adhere to a pedagogy that takes into account the human fabric and not only the content of a set program of study.

The link between relaxation and vigilance

According to yoga, concentration is an illusory tool unless it is associated with a certain threshold of calm.

The West often confuses attention and tension; but researchers, thanks to the recent studies on stress, have begun to realize that effective activity is significantly linked to relaxed vigilance. To prove it, the latest pedagogical thinking emphasizes that a certain degree of awareness associated with a state of relaxation unites all the favorable factors for studying. We can conclude from this, that it is less effective to strain yourself toward a set goal than it is to relax yourself into it.

The advantage of this state of peaceful awareness is that it revives the pleasure of learning. When a whole class experiences this state of consciousness in silence, an intense joy invigorates attention and stimulates memory. These techniques for accelerated learning highlight the need to empty the inner space in order to clarify the emerging ideas.

EXERCISE 15 — THE WIND THAT CHASES THE CLOUDS

Starting Position

Students are seated comfortably, eyes shut and relaxed. Their books are already opened to the day's lesson.

Procedure

- Feel your feet on the ground, your buttocks on the chair, and your whole body in the space of the classroom.

- Become aware of the stillness of your body; listen to the sound of your breath. You will be doing an exercise that helps chase away fatigue and all anxieties that prevent you from feeling the sunshine within you.

- First, visualize gray and black clouds in the sky. They represent your worries, your fears, your boredom and your fatigue.

- With each exhalation, you can hear within yourself a rising breeze that chases the clouds. Quickly, see a small blue space being created among the clouds. This strip of blue sky becomes bigger with each breath. I am going to leave you to continue chasing these gray clouds *(pause)*.

- Now, your inner sky is totally blue and the sun is shining bright. Thus when you are happy, the sun shines within you. With every inhalation, breathe in sunlight; and with every exhalation, spread its joy and light to your heart and in your head. You are feeling good *(pause)*.

- Think of a time when you were happy to learn something new. Recreate this warm feeling now. There is sunshine in your heart *(pause)*. You are in this happy state of mind to begin the lesson.

- Become aware of the contact of your body with the chair, with the floor, feel the presence of your friends in the class who have all, just like you, seen the blue sky within. Open your eyes now and look at your book.

Link with Tradition

This exercise is drawn from *Dharana*.

Effects

This exercise considerably changes the atmosphere of the class. It is a very powerful method of purifying the spirit.

It combines respiration and visualization of archetypal images. It has a powerful effect on the imagination of children. They instantly and straightforwardly understand the importance of a peaceful inner state.

Best Use of the Exercise

This exercise is especially good at the beginning of a lesson, particularly when students are tired and low in spirits. It is an excellent exercise to do during the winter season when the daylight hours are few.

EXERCISE 16 — THE POINT AND THE CIRCLE

Preparation

The students are seated, backs straight. The teacher draws a colored point on the blackboard.

Procedure

- Raise your index finger to the level of the eyes, around thirty centimeters from the face and in the direction of the point that I have just drawn on the blackboard. Now look at both the tip of your finger and at the point on the blackboard at the same time.

- Become aware of your breath. Inhaling, look at the tip of your finger and while exhaling fix your gaze on the point. Breathe very slowly and notice the difference of the visual plane between the finger and the point. Continue *(long pause)*.

- Lower the finger and close your eyes; focus your attention on the inner space behind your closed eyes. See a point. Maybe it is the image of the point that I have drawn on the board or maybe it is the tip of your finger .... If not, create a point and visualize it. Keep your face calm and relaxed.

- Observe the color of the point and see it becoming progressively bigger. It is the image of your concentration. It is growing into a luminous sphere that lights up your entire brain. You are happy to be able to concentrate and are ready to work.

- Let go of all these images. Notice the light coming through your eyelids; feel your body on the chair. Bring yourself back to the present, open your eyes and look at your book.

Link with Tradition

This exercise deals with the interplay between the yoga notions of external *tratak*, leading to *antar-tratak* or internal focus.

Best Use of the Exercise

It is good to use this exercise whenever the mental energy in class has been dissipated, i.e. after a recess or playtime. It gives excellent results before a written test.

Observations

This is the same type of exercise as the one of re-centering through eyesight. It gives a child the opportunity to visualize concretely through a tactile image and emphasizes the important concept of concentration.

EXERCISE 17—A CHAIN OF WORDS

Starting Position

The students are seated comfortably, their elbows on the table. They can eventually be holding their heads in their hands. The eyes are shut.

Procedure

- Become aware of your position: your feet on the ground *(pause)*, your buttocks on the chair *(pause)*. Become aware of your whole body *(pause)*. Now, I will name different parts of your body and I want you to repeat mentally the name at the same time as you feel each part:

    1. Right foot, right leg, right side of the chest, right arm, right hand.

    2. Left foot, left leg, left side of the chest, left arm, left hand.

    3. The whole back. The whole head. The whole front of the body. The whole body completely still *(pause)*. Feel your calm breath.

- I will give you a series of words; they are part of the lesson. Visualize the image of the word and repeat it mentally: horse … farm…dog…hen…meadow … milk…cow-bells.

- Re-visualize these 7 images in the correct order *(pause)*. Now, I will call out the list of words one more time. Make a mental note of the words that you have forgotten. The teacher repeats the words *(pause)*. Now, re-visualize these 7 images one more time *(pause)*. Good. Tomorrow, I will add three new words to the list.

- Become aware of your body sitting on the chair, in the class. Open your eyes. Write down these words in your notebook.

Link with Tradition

Dharana develops the ability to visualize images clearly and to re-hear sounds mentally.

Effects

This exercise develops a strong memory.

Best Use of the Exercise

This kind of practice can be incorporated as part of the lesson.

Observations

This technique can be performed with many variations. One of the most interesting ones for training memory consists of remembering the list while adding two to three more words every lesson. After a few months, the students will be able to remember a string of images so long that the teacher will have to make note of them beforehand in her planning book!

To develop the children's creativity, we can ask students to combine certain images to form stories that they can then recount, write out or draw at the end of the exercise.

This is an excellent method for teaching vocabulary in a foreign language class.

Pleasure pays off

One of the great guiding principles in education is that of joyful effort. The exercises that we propose here are both rigorous and fun, which might seem paradoxical to Westerners like us. Finding pleasure in work! This is where the shoe pinches. Haven't we been condemned to work by the sweat of our brow since Adam and Eve bit into the apple? In that fateful moment, they were cursed to toil on earth; they and all generations thereafter would have to suffer pain and boredom. Since then, Paradise at school, like Eden on Earth, is over!

Well think again! We do not believe pleasure to be the enemy of effective work. On the contrary, and this for three reasons:

- First, pleasure does not run counter to discipline.

- Second, a feeling of well being improves memory; this has been proved scientifically.

- Third, finding pleasure in work, is a guarantee for good physical and mental health.

Ask yourself this question, "Would you be taken aback if your child were to tell you that she enjoys studying?" Mark your response:

YES or NO

If you said YES: be careful! You carry all the weight of Adam and Eve's mistake. Let the sun shine within you!

If you said NO: bravo, you are mature! The fruits of enjoyable labor are no longer forbidden to you. Enjoy them!

PART TWO

FINDING DIRECTION
IN LIFE

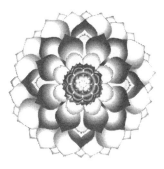

A constructive search, far removed from Science Fiction

The renewed interest in body fitness has played a major role in the fashion of returning to natural ways. However, staying in good shape alone does not seem to some of us to be the ultimate goal. Many of us, eager to go further, have set out on an inner search. Like salmon that surmount all natural and man-made barriers in their quest of origin, many people today are seeking the source of a vibrant reality.

In this search, they are often guided by one tradition or another, be it from the East or the West. Yoga is at the base of most of these. Its advantage is that it comes to us as a complete science, starting with the physical body and progressing in measured steps to the inner core. This nucleus gives us direction in life, even when all else fails. This slow and sure unfolding of the inner self makes any recourse to drugs unnecessary.

During a visit to America, we were surprised to discover some students being handed prescribed tranquilizers in their school on their way to class! We thought at the time, in 1974, that this was an isolated case which had its place within the context of a few big American cities. Today this practice of tranquilizing schoolchildren by means of pharmaceuticals, which seemed so unthinkable to us then, has found its way everywhere.

Multiple investigations in all industrialized countries have shown that one student out of two take analgesics more or less regularly. In fact, it appears that high school young people are among the largest consumers of sleeping pills and tranquilizers. Their schools are not the only culprits. Their parents, too, have given them a taste for calming drugs and quick fixes since the time they were toddlers.

The overuse of these new types of pabulum should have put adult parents on their guard. Would their young people have developed such habits had it not been for their own example? Or is this not the logical consequence of a way of life, founded on a certain vision of the world?

Our western society seems to be confronting the ultimate consequence of materialism, which pushes us to look for the solution to all our ailments on the surface.

At the same time we are witnessing a huge explosion of interest in Eastern wisdom. We hear talk of the renaissance of yoga in the West. A current of great force seems to be carrying the yoga movement, and with good reason. Instead of rejecting the senses it tends to restructure them.

When the yogi thinks of energy

If there is a capital that deserves to be managed well it is the energy of life, manifest in young people. But what do we see? An energy which explodes in youth and gets blown away by the prevailing winds of puberty! What then has Yoga to say about this? A lot! And this, because the subject matter concerns the correct management of an energy oriented toward the success of an enterprise none other than our own life. Listen to us. It is not only a matter of succeeding on intellectual, athletic or professional planes, but in every aspect of our personality. You may have already noticed that some people will succeed extremely well in their outward careers yet fail pitifully in their private lives, or vise versa. While still others, who seem to 'have everything to be happy about', are plagued by depression. These are signs that the craftsmen of 'success' have forgotten to deal with the essential.

Perhaps they would have done better had they followed the

advice of Emerson to the seekers of gold in the 19th century, "Hitch your wagon to a star!" It is all fine and good to lead dynamic and adventurous lives, provided we point our compass in the right direction!

The young generation does not lack energy, but self knowledge that will lead them to identify what it is that they really want. It is only when we know ourselves truly, that we can begin to minimize the occasions where we squander our energy. We must learn to save our inner resources, so that we can give the best of ourselves.

With the multiple diversions of our consumer-oriented society and pulled this way and that by false needs and insipid pleasures, our young people are ill-treated and disappointed by school. They graduate, understanding neither their responsibilities nor their role in society. Why should they bother to learn? Becoming cynical and with a feeling of being defeated in advance, they function without any confidence in the future and, even worse, in themselves. We might refer to them as "maladjusted". But, what kind of scholastic guidance can we give to "re-adjust" these young people onto the high road to success?

The way to "re-adjustment"

Experience demonstrates daily that young people have an unquenchable thirst to understand the laws of life, values far higher than those of consumerism alone. Our educational system seems to put all its energy into tearing young people away from the quest for self that would spontaneously lead them a little closer to their inner joy. Must we confine them to the situation of someone who, having lost the keys to his house, stands and gesticulates furiously outside his door for want of a locksmith?

Bringing yoga into the classroom makes it possible to re-establish equilibrium by introducing the forgotten element in our teaching: that of inner life, of silence and of **awareness.**

73

Although these moments are short, they are all the more precious. They make it possible for us to avoid the ill effects of the many disturbances that surround us. At a time when talk about failure in our schools is on everyone's lips, these moments of re-centering will help us to stabilize nerves and to cope with class work. They will prepare students for intense periods of study and will invigorate their health.

To strive towards a new school 'culture' is a matter of utmost necessity. One could compare today's child to a rocky ground where we sow select seeds – our seemingly marvelous school programs - without taking into consideration the topsoil which is required so that the seeds can take root and grow. Tied up in knots by stress, the gray matter of the child's brain is nothing more than a sterile heap of rubble. Let us act now to avoid the waste of our life force.

The motto of all education can be summed up in one word, ***recentering.***

This is precisely the aim of the exercises presented in the following pages. They are concerned with reconditioning that faculty, so essential for mental health, ***concentration.***

Yoga, which has been involved in this domain for a long time, provides us with an excellent metaphor and tool, ***the mandala.***

1

Concentration —
The Barometer of Energy
Four States of Concentration

Yoga provides us with a means to diagnose the quality of our energy. We need only observe the quality of our concentration, or how well we pay attention, to know how energetic we are. Successful teaching is based precisely on this criterion. The teachers constantly ask their pupils to pay attention. Yoga provides them means to achieve this. We all agree that a good student should be capable of focusing his attention at will on a specific point, or on a given piece of work.

Below are the criteria for an energy diagnosis in function of the attention level in class. *(See drawings on page 76.)*

1. Lethargic Attention

This child is in need of awakening exercises more than relaxation exercises. We call him a "nice" child but he's asleep. He does not seem to be interested in anything.

2. Fluctuating Attention

This child is our typical "agitator". Whereas in the preceding case, we could infer rather than conclude a take-over by the parasympathetic system, here the sympathetic nervous system is over-active. This type of child needs calming exercises. Training him in relaxation techniques will help him a lot. This child is inquisitive but only superficially, interested but not for long. He wastes his overall energy.

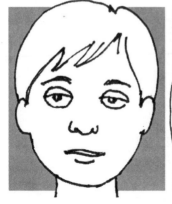

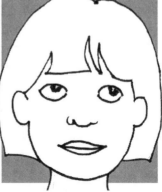

1. Lethargic Attention *2. Fluctuating Attention*

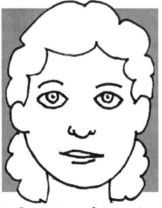

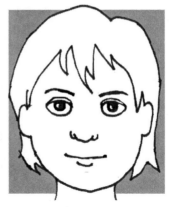

3. Concentrated Attention *4. Perfect attention*

3. Concentrated Attention

This kind of attention is found in our 'well behaved' children. They have the advantage of a good neurological-vegetative balance which facilitates their learning. They know how to work consistently. They listen well and respond correctly. This profile can hide a negative aspect if the child is a conformist or a creature of habit. In fact, concentration and inner calm may go hand in hand with enthusiasm and creativity, two necessary qualities for a balanced child.

4. Perfect attention

It is the most complete form among those which we have just described, but also the rarest. It is seen in children gifted with an exceptional level of intelligence and capacity for concentration. Attentiveness comes naturally to them. We may observe that these four faces express the various levels of intensity of the attitudes of the same child or group of children in the course of a day.

Thus, on Monday morning, in the start hour, relaxation is not usually needed because 'the primordial energy' is still *asleep* (1). The ends of the morning and afternoon correspond to the *fluctuating type* (2). The mid-morning on Tuesday for example, might correspond to the *concentrated type* (3). Lastly comes that blessed moment when the whole group participates in an activity which is highly stimulating for the personality. A special connection is established with the proposed assignment. We might observe in this situation a *connected type* (4).

These attention levels based on *gunas*, which have been identified since time immemorial, constitute benchmarks that are valuable today. They allow the teacher to estimate the available energy in the class at any given time of the day and to adjust the lesson plan accordingly, choosing from among the appropriate exercises, ones that will act to invigorate, relax or balance. Once the diagnosis has been made, all you need is the prescribed remedy. Let us discuss some of the choices.

EXERCISE 18 — A GAME OF LISTENING AND SILENCE

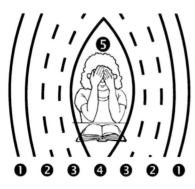

1. Most distant sounds

2. Sounds immediately outside the classroom

3. Three little sounds inside the classroom

4. Music in decrescendo

5. Sound of the breath

Procedure

- The children are in their seats, elbows on the table, the hands cupped over their eyes. Their books are open, lying on the table, to the page of the lesson for the day. The teacher gives instructions according to the level of comprehension and age of the class:

- "Let's relax. Listen to the sounds from the street." *(Pause for 30 to 40 seconds.)*

- "Listen to the sounds from the courtyard." *(Pause for 30 to 40 seconds.)*

- "Listen to the sounds in the classroom. Notice that we are not immersed into complete silence. *(Pause 30 to 40 seconds.)*

- "In the classroom right now thanks to you, there is silence. You are still and listening. I will deliberately make 3 small, very small noises, one after the other."

> *(1st Noise: light crumpling of paper.)*
> *(2nd noise: clicking of a ballpoint pen)*
> *(3rd noise: light tapping on the desk)*

- "Mentally try to recall them in order now." *(Pause.)*

- "Good. You are all listening. I will play some music but, pay close attention. Open your ears. I will play it low, very low." *(Music played at very low volume.)*

- "When you do not hear it any more, you will hear the quietest rustle of all, that of your breath going in and out of your nostrils."*(Pause.)*

- "Feel your breath which is your life force, dilating your rib cage and filling and expanding your back." *(Pause.)*

- "Breathe more deeply now. Listen to the sound it makes, like the noise of the sea and the waves. Count the waves." *(Pause.)*

- "Feel the breath gently in your nostrils." *(Pause.)*

- "Remember the little sounds I made that you heard earlier." *(Pause.)*

- "Now, listen to the noises on the street." *(Pause.)*

- "Listen to the music again. Feel your body on the chair, your elbows on the table. Gently take your hands away from your eyes while keeping your eyes closed. See the light filtering through your eyelids. Keep your eyes shut and listen or open your eyes and follow the text on the page if you prefer, as I read..."

Link with Tradition

This exercise is *Antar Mauna*, one of the fundamental exercises of *Raja Yoga*, where you listen to external noises as a way to attain silence.

Recommendation

Instead of noises, you can use music that you gradually

decrease in volume, inviting students to try and catch the least audible sound.

Best Use of the Exercise

Can be done either after exercises or after a recreational period to assist in the transition to intellectual work.

Effects

This exercise is excellent for re-focusing children's attention through listening. It can be adapted in any number of ways to suit lessons which require auditory attention, for example, reading aloud the text of a lesson.

EXERCISE 19 — THE MAGIC CIRCLE,

Development of Visual Memory

The technique of concentration on a point - called *tratak* in yoga - can be carried out at the beginning of a class in which the sense of sight will be used. We invite you to try this exercise now:

- Prepare a text for reading; it can be the continuation of this chapter.

- Straighten your back, and then become aware of the parts of your body in contact with the ground or the chair on which you are seated – soles of your feet, your buttocks. Now, relax your face, forehead, eyebrows, jaws.

- Gaze for 50 seconds at the center of the wheel shown on the following page. There should be no tension in your face. Simply tell yourself, "My eyes remain fixed on the small central point without moving a millimeter."

- Inhale. Now while exhaling, move your eyes suddenly to

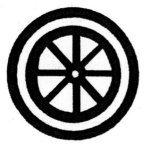

the right and onto the small black spot. You will see an after image. Focus in on the point. If nothing comes, blink a little.

- Close your eyes, relax your eyelids and once again focus on the after image in the inner space. It will disappear little by little. If you do not see anything, just watch the space behind the forehead.

- Keep the face relaxed and once again focus your attention on the outer environment. Feel your buttocks on the chair, the soles of your feet on the ground.

- Open your eyes gradually and look at the text and begin to read it. Become aware of the quality of your concentration.

A doctor studies the effects of yoga in class

The body and the mind effect each other. A good example of this is reflected in the old saying that an irascible and melancholic person is of a "bile humor". This expression reflects ancient and medieval physiology, which defined humors as related to one of our four body fluids: blood, phlegm and choler (yellow) and black bile (from the Latin 'bilis'). Western man has observed since antiquity that our mental state has physiological effects. The following experiment conducted in school shows us just how true this is.

Doctor Françoise Herreman, a cardiologist and specialist in yoga, having learned of our research into yoga at school, suggested that we study how fluctuations in the attention level of the children affected their heartbeats.

The heart is an organ that receives impulses from the entire body. When the body – including the brain - is calm, the heart is calm too. On the other hand, if the body is agitated and the mind distracted, the heart is likewise affected.

The Holter, a battery-powered apparatus, the size of a small tape recorder, was equipped with electrodes that were placed on the chests of several children. The children therefore could continue their lessons in a completely normal manner. (This technique of measurement is usually employed in sport medicine to monitor an athlete's performance. It is also used in aeronautics to monitor test pilots but we shall return to this later.)

Continuing with our experiment, the heart does not always beat at the same speed. Even when you are seated and seemingly motionless the heart demonstrates irregular activity. The Holter registers cardio variability by means of computer imaging; it furnishes us with a picture of this biological fluctuation, so necessary to life. We therefore ran tests on an English language class and had students perform yogic exercises for concentration.

Our findings showed a great deal of variation in the heartbeats before the beginning of class and at times when there is a change of activity. On the other hand, when the teacher asked the students to concentrate on a given point, with eyes open and then closed, we found that the cardio activity was perfectly balanced. All heartbeats occurred at the same frequency for the duration of the exercise. It was as if the heart had become quiet in order to "hear" the brain.

In other words, *mental dissipation has the power to distract the heart, and undoubtedly disrupts other organs as well.*

2

Keep cool...... ok, but how?

Under a calm exterior, a storm rages

While testing, we found that under their apparent calm, the hearts of fighter pilots often hid enormous stress. Holter readings of pilots' heart beats have shown that in some cases their heart rates rose dangerously during the flight. The possibility of a heart attack in the air sometimes forces them to stop flying for safety reasons.

Learning to control one's nerves is important and we consider this to be especially true in the area of children's education.

These experiments make us question the meaning of our commonly-held concept of self control. If a violent effort to hide our feelings and reactions is required, it will only increase stress and force our body/mind to redirect the repressed impulses elsewhere in the system.

In the same way, an iron discipline imposed by a tyrannical teacher will have almost the same effect. The class will seem so good that you can hear a pin drop! But what about the storm within the brain and the racing heart within the rib cage? Must we force this terrible strain on frozen bodies and on tongues tied in knots by fear? The ideal which yoga proposes is a sense of confidence which evolves through self-discipline.

One day a refrigerator breaks down and a red indicator lights up. The owner calls in a repairman who tries to find out what is wrong to no avail. Finally, worn out and pressed for time, he simply severs the wire from the red indicator. No more symptoms! The problem is solved but the refrigerator still does not work. In our system of education we are all too often more concerned with putting out the red indicator than coming to grips with the real problem.

Violence, a short-circuit of energy

The sages have always said, and we know it to be true, that energy which is not directed towards a higher goal is destined to tumble down with a great crash. The violence that we see today in our classrooms is an unconscious revolt against the ideal of materialism that society offers to young people. Excessive consumption awakens their animal instincts.

What distinguishes men from other animals if not the capacity to refrain from their savage urges? Today, we know that this faculty is situated in the frontal lobe of the brain, responsible for control and decision making. We can speak of it as being a sort of 'control panel' in the brain. Have you ever noticed the narrowness of the skull of a prehistoric man compared to that of a human being today? If so, you will easily understand the importance of this zone of control which, by widening, shows the direction of human evolution.

Yogis have always placed a great value on gaining awareness of the space behind the forehead. Based on the latest research as much as on yoga, we can state the following law:

Any impulse that becomes conscious releases one from uncontrolled fury.

This is an eminently human ability. It is important that a child learns to think before he acts, so that the consequences of his instinctive actions may first be visualized on the inner screen (forehead area) of his conscience. It may be no more than a split-second period of awareness, but a decisive one. We observe action and we react as witnesses. Popular wisdom correctly advises us to think before we act. This latency period, however short, is necessary in order for us to defuse the harmful effects of fear and aggressiveness. We believe that a systematic practice in self control would have a great impact on reducing juvenile violence and delinquency. So we can see how important it is that these yoga exercises for awareness and self control should begin very early in the child's life. From six and seven years of age, from the time a child starts primary school, it is necessary for him to be made aware of correct posture and breathing which over time will lead him to observe his inner states and develop self knowledge.

Recommendation

As often as possible teach the child to visualize whatever action you suggest he should do before he actually does it.

EXERCISE 20 — A MEASURED ACTION
Procedure

- Bring the chair close to the desk, back straight, arms bent, elbows on the table. The hands are relaxed with palms facing the table.
- The hands are completely relaxed, this is level zero. Then follow through the 4 levels below, beginning with the right hand.

1. Visualization of the movement beforehand

- Let's visualize in our head the movement that we will perform in a few seconds. Like a camera that is projecting a film in slow motion, you are going to close your right hand very slowly into a fist. (figure ①)

2. Start of the movement

- Bend your fingers in towards the palms. (figure ②)

3. Completion of the movement

- Without haste and strain, let the fingers touch your palm and fold into a fist. (figure ③)

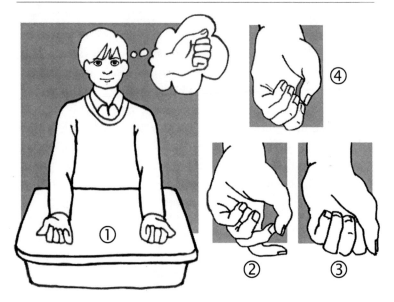

4. Tighten the fist while inhaling

- Hold your breath for 2 seconds. Then on the exhale, open your hand slowly, without haste and strain. *(figure ④)*

- Repeat these 4 steps once again with the left hand and once with both hands together.

Link with Tradition

This exercise is *vinyasa*, which means "gradual effort".

Effects

This exercise in differential relaxation brings into play the frontal zones of the brain cortex where the centers of discernment and decision making are located. The step by step process accustoms children to introduce a pause between impulse and action. The distinction of the 4 levels allows the awakening of consciousness in two essential phases : (1) the project of action with its preparation and (2) the phase of the action itself. Thus, the children learn mastery over themselves. Many studies have shown how important it is for the brain to refrain from its animal reactions. Exercises of this type are excellent for preventing awkward movements and uncontrolled aggressive behaviors.

Best Use of the Exercise

- Before a relaxation exercise, whether the relaxation relates to the hands only or to other parts of the body
- After an exercise where the children have written or drawn a lot
- After a period of recreation
- After a period of recess
- Generally speaking, when students are tense and noisy

Variation

This exercise can be done using the lower limbs or other parts of the body, such as the face, and even using the whole body.

Remark

With right-handers it is better to start with the right hand, with left-handers, the left. When doing the exercise as a group, it is better to have the same instruction for everyone in order to avoid confusion.

Enhancing 'Presence'

Psychologists all agree that the act of teaching wears a person out. In other words, one's nervous system takes a beating in our usual teacher-student relationship. From the teacher's point of view, the practice of yoga is like a life buoy or a whiff of pure oxygen that carries them over the troubled waters of their trade. It is also a valuable tool in instances where the strain of daily events takes its toll on school life. There is one thing a teacher needs more than anything else, a set of strong nerves.

It is common knowledge that just because someone is a great thinker or an expert in his field, does not mean that he will automatically know how to transmit that knowledge to others as a teacher. For that, it is necessary that he be gifted with that little extra "je ne sais quoi" that makes a good teacher, what we sometimes call presence, that special charm which some teachers seem to lack. But wait a minute, the situation isn't hopeless. Presence can be learned.

This is a true story, told by a teacher we know. One day, as a teaching inspector was paying a surprise visit in her class, she became so overcome with fear that she lost the train of thought of what she was trying to explain to her pupils, which resulted in a situation you can imagine. It went so bad that she broke down in tears, abandoning the lesson that she had, as usual, carefully prepared. Afterwards, the inspector commented to her, "Mademoiselle, you are too emotional, you should do yoga!" The young woman recorded these words in her memory. She took them to be more a criticism than a suggestion. She repeated them to her fellow teachers when they met in conference. One of her colleagues, instead of laughing at her, pointed out the wisdom of the inspector's advice and succeeded in convincing her to practice yoga. Two years later, the same inspector returned to her class and noted a spectacular improvement in the lesson and the demeanor of the teacher. Now, sure of herself, the teacher explained, "On your advice, I started practicing yoga!" Strangely enough, the inspector was surprised by this remark because she no longer had any recollection of it. The inspector had shot out this derisive suggestion on the spur of the moment as a joke, inspired by hearsay, no doubt. But this little phrase had sown a seed of wisdom which in two years time had borne fruit.

This anecdote catches our attention because it provides a real example, in time and space, of what can happen when you practice what we preach. By continued practice, it is quite possible for you to change to the point where your inner growth becomes manifest outwardly in a very positive way.

This personal work on self-improvement involves two aspects:

- Firstly, daily personal hygiene: the maintenance of good

physical condition enables us to preserve an upright attitude, in keeping with our noble profession.

- Secondly, the effective techniques of self-observation allow the development of a witness attitude. This is the Trojan horse that enters the place so well defended by our rigid armor. The luminous arrows of the awakening consciousness eliminate, one by one, our deep-rooted defects that so often irritate those around us.

The practice of yoga gives us a new vision of ourselves, that enables us to step back and perceive ourselves otherwise.

EXERCISE 21 — THE WITNESS

An exercise designed for teachers.

Starting position

In a seated position, back straight, eyes closed, face and body relaxed, preferably after a *hatha-yoga* practice, become aware of the stillness of the body and the surrounding sounds.

Procedure

- Focus your attention on the space behind the forehead - the inner space – and allow any thoughts that enter to flow freely. By "thoughts", we mean any perceptions, image or feeling which might occur, including whatever ideas might happen to cross your mind. These are vagabonds. Allow them to pass by, without losing your attitude of witness and without "coloring" them with emotions. If the thoughts are merry, do not enjoy yourself; if they are sad, do not become sad. Stay neutral and attentive. Watch the empty spaces between the thoughts when the flow slows down, maybe due to your observation. On the other hand, if they stream by, one after the other, notice the absence of a "blank" between them.

(Pause.)

- Think about events from your daily life. Recall each activity: leaving your house, entering the classroom, running errands. Keep yourself removed from the image, as if you were watching a film. Above all, do not judge yourself. Set aside your faculties of analysis. The result will be that much better.

- Bring your attention back to your breath, your body and to external noises.

Link with Tradition

This practice is called *Antar Mouna*, the practice of 'inner silence'.

Though we have given you a classic exercise practiced preferably while being seated, back upright, in a favorable environment, it is possible to do it in any number of positions—seated or standing, walking or riding in a car, and so on. In short, any circumstance in life lends itself to this exercise. Some of us like to do it systematically before we begin to teach, because we have realized that being mindful of our inner state has a calming effect which is beneficial to us at work. This exercise also seems to have a contagious effect on the extraneous noise level of the students, which decreases in volume, as if our inner attitude were spreading out into the classroom. *Silence begets silence.*

3

Mandala, a Guiding Force as Old as the World

Universality of mandala

Have you ever noticed how, in times of crises, we long for some anchor, some center point? We can see a parallel to this replicated spontaneously everywhere in nature. It is called *mandala.*

What is meant by *mandala?* This word of Sanskrit origin means 'circle' and more generally it indicates a geometric figure organized around a center, comprised of squares, triangles or something else. Let us keep to the Sanskrit word *mandala* without translating it, because its scope goes far beyond that of a simple circular figure. In spite of its name, mandala is not restricted to Tibet or India; it is universal.

A glance at art books of the many civilizations of the world is enough to verify mandala's omnipresence. People pour much love into them. Look at the pyramids, Tibetan tankas, African and American totems, the rose windows of our cathedrals, the keltic triskells of Brittany and all kinds of coats of arms.

The world over, it guides research and creations, whether scientific or artistic.

The mandala—a secret code of nature

The American Indians used to set up their 'tepees' in circular encampments. This tradition calls to mind the words of a Sioux chief:

"The power of the world always appears in a circle and everything tries to be round. The sun and the moon rise and set in the form of a circle, even the seasons complete a cycle and return to where they started from. The life of man is a circle, from childhood to childhood. And so it is wherever the Great Spirit is at work."

This force can be seen in all of nature in those perfect examples of mandalas which we call flowers, butterflies and trees. Rumi, the great Sufi poet, said that if you open a grain of sand, you discover the sun and the planets around it. This is exactly what physicists have shown to be true, in the infinitely small as well as in the infinitely large. Electrons move around the nuclear core making arabesques, just as the movement of our own life is made up of the eternal dancing of the mandalas within us.

Perhaps the mandala contains the very secret to the encoding of information at a molecular level. The structure of DNA represented in its spiral form is an authentic mandala.

The mandala—a welcoming abode

This dwelling from which men of all times have drawn new energy is built around the simple and precise principles of architecture. Traditionally, we find:

1. The center

It can be a two-dimensional point or a three-dimensional horizontal or vertical axis, like the spinal column for example, pillar of the human body.

It is from this center that space organizes itself. Cocteau said that, "The center is the place where speed sleeps on the spot." It is indeed the focal point of condensed energy, the symbol of one's inner being.

Our language is revealing. A person who is not doing well in life is said to be "disoriented" or "beside himself" whereas someone who is well balance seems centered.

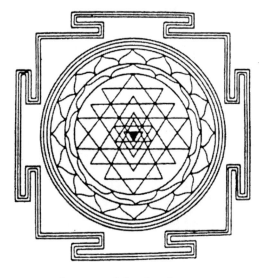

Indian Mandala, the Shri Yantra.

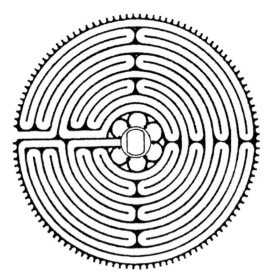

Western Mandala,
the Labyrinth of Chartres Cathedral

93

2. Complementary parts

Notice that the forms and the colors laid out around the center are not strictly symmetrical. Though we may not be aware of it at first glance, closer observation will reveal subtle variations in the apparent symmetry of the elements. The secret of the deep harmony of a mandala lies not in symmetry, that impoverishes and freezes, but rather in complementarity.

3. An enclosure and doors.

The traditional mandala presents the central figure flanked by four doors cut at each side in a square.

The enclosed square is the image of both protection and welcome. A door stands either 'open' or 'shut'. If shut, it symbolizes an enclosed space where energies are re-composing. Thus, during sleep, our senses withdraw into the inside letting deep consciousness replenish the strength that has been depleted by the days activities.

When the door is open, a new dynamic is let in, one which is receptive to interaction and leads transformation. Thus mandalas are powerful tools for evolution.

Above all, let us underline that they symbolize an essential factor of everything in existence—organization. They are an expression of the path from hurly-burly to order, from chaos to cosmos.

The carry over of mandala into the third millennium

Omnipresent throughout the civilizations of the past, does the mandala still have a place in today's world in the midst of advancing technologies or is it doomed to fall into oblivion in favor of the new computer king? At the turn of the twenty-first century, many wise people have already sent out repeated warnings: man needs to uphold his inner values against the invasion of enervating machines. We do not mean that all the blame should be laid on the triumph of information technology, which has brought benefits to the individual and society as a whole. But we should be wary, lest the human brain itself become programmed. Will we be reduced to mere numbers? Will we become like robots, good only for duplicating ourselves in endless series? What would become of creative genius in a world where everything is pre-planned? Some will say that this is taking things too far, but only time will tell. Certainly we have reached the point where our efforts are almost solely applied to developing the intellect, which is already over-sized. Should we avoid this by calling on some para-psychological power at the risk of losing our sanity?

No, this is not an acceptable option.

Rather, let us stimulate creative intuition through the use of these diagrams of concentrated energy known as mandalas. These figures have a great affinity with the ways in which the brain operates. Isn't our brain like a kaleidoscope, where under the influence of the vital force coiled within us, the permutations and ceaseless combinations of geometrical forms burst forth with all the inventions that aid the progress of mankind? In other words the mandala symbolizes all creation, past, present and future. This is why the contemplation of famous forms like the *Shri Yantra* and the Labyrinth of Chartres stimulates in us new thoughts and reorients us toward a constructive goal. Such is the yogic theory of perception, which is now being proved by modern research. Undoubtedly, the mandala still has its role to play in the third millennium. Leave it in place; this old guide may well prove irreplaceable.

Testing a mandala

If you give a pencil to a three-year-old, he will immediately start making circles. Any pre-school teacher has observed this natural reaction on the part of young toddlers. It highlights the irresistible fascination of even very young children for mandalas. This instinct can be put to advantage in helping them to learn better. Our experience and that of all our teaching colleagues from every academic discipline who, like us, have used mandalas in class, concur. The mandala—children like the term—is immensely popular both with the teachers who propose them and with the students who appreciate the infinite play of its forms and colors. The children's richly colored drawings of circles decorate the classroom walls and lend themselves to all kinds of inventions and explosions of creativity.

The olive in the middle of the dish.

Notice how culinary art attaches great importance to the presentation of food. Watch the lady of the house preparing canapés. What she is actually making, instinctively, are small tasty mandalas. This observation brings us to the heart of our subject.

One reads in scholarly texts by dietitians about the importance of experiencing pleasure at the sight of food; it stimulates the secretion of gastric juices and digestive enzymes. So we can begin by saying that mandala participates in the health of the stomach. The olive in the middle of the canapé or the chocolate chip in the center of a cookie is the finishing touch which helps us to better assimilate food.

But what does all this fine cookery have to do with school? Knowledge is better digested by the brain when it is well presented. The mandala appeals strongly to the minds of children, young and old. It is a remarkable element which sharpens their love of learning, even for the most abstract and unappealing subjects.

Just because the mandala has a strong impact on learning does not mean that it is a panacea. It is not necessary to serve it at every meal or to make of it the only item on the menu.

Let's not overdo a good thing; variety in good measure is the spice of life in the classroom as well as at table.

Use the mandala as a learning tool.

EXERCISE 22 — THE MANDALA OF ASSOCIATIONS

Stage 1
Constructing a mandala

From a given word students must look for all associations that come to mind. This exercise can be done individually or in a group. One must not force these thoughts but let the associated ideas emerge spontaneously, as in the example below.

Beginning with the word 'sun'.

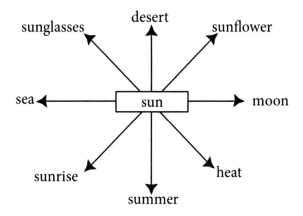

Now your turn, beginning with the word 'tree'.

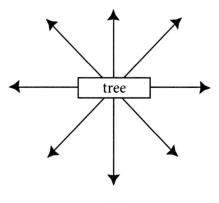

Stage 2

External concentration; reading of the words around the mandala

Here is the transcription of the exercise, the way it is described to students, starting with the word 'sun':

"Fix your eyes on the center of the mandala and mentally say the word 'sun' *(brief pause).*

"Follow the arrow with your gaze up to the word 'desert' and say it to yourselves, 'desert' *(brief pause).*

"Return towards the center 'sun' and repeat this word mentally *(brief pause).* Set out again towards the periphery up to the related word 'sunflower' which you will repeat silently *(brief pause).*

"Return towards 'sun' and mentally repeat it *(brief pause).*

"Move the eyes along the arrow towards the word 'moon'. At your own pace, continue this to and fro movement between the center and each of the 8 peripheral associations in a clockwise direction, until you have made one full rotation *(long pause).*

"Close your eyes, relax your eyelids and cup your hands over them. Notice how your head is a 'darkroom' *(pause).*

"Remove your hands from your eyes and become slowly aware again of where you are; feel your buttocks on the chair, the soles of your feet on the ground.

"Now open your eyes."

Variation of stage 2

This exercise can be synchronized with the breath; exhale while moving the gaze towards the peripheral association and inhale while returning towards the center. The mental repetition must be done at that brief moment when you stop inhaling, lungs full (sun) and exhaling, lungs empty (the association).

We invite you to carry out this exercise yourselves, starting from the word 'tree'.

Stage 3

Mental concentration; visualization

Here is the transcription of the exercise as given to students once they have learned the associations by heart:

Preparation: "Close your eyes, relax your eyelids and focus your attention on your spine. Feel the soles of your feet on the ground *(pause)*, your buttocks on the chair *(pause)*, your breathing from the abdomen *(pause)*. Become aware of the inner space, behind your forehead. It is permeated with a pale luminosity filtering through your closed eyelids *(pause)*.

The Actual Practice: "Now, mentally go through the associations in this manner. When you say the word, see the 'image' of the word appear in your mind. Remember that after each association you return to the center according to this sequence: sun - the first association - sun - the second association and so on with quite a fast rhythm. With every pronunciation an image is projected on your mental screen. If nothing comes, do not worry; move on to the next one. Keep your face relaxed *(long pause)*.

Return: "Give up your review of the inner space and of the associations and become aware again of the luminosity behind your forehead *(pause)*. Observe the passage of air through your nostrils *(pause)*. Move your attention back down along the spine: notice your abdominal breathing, feel the contact of your buttocks with the chair, the soles of your feet on the ground *(pause)*. Move your toes, as if you wished to dig them into the ground so that you feel well rooted *(pause)*. Now finish and open your eyes."

Again. we invite you to carry out this exercise yourselves starting from the word 'tree'.

Observations

1. This practice of association can be adapted to suit almost every circumstance. For example, it can be used for finding words in order to enrich the vocabulary. The comparisons can then become a search for synonyms, for words of the same family, for adjectives characterizing a concept or simply, as above, for free associations. Associations can be used to describe the properties of one or another geometrical figure or to find out the causes and consequences of an historical event, and so on...

2. This exercise develops memory and concentration.

3. By combining repetition (mental) and visualization, this practice mobilizes both hemispheres of the brain at the same time. The center of language is located in the left hemisphere, whereas mental imagery is situated in the right hemisphere.

4. As you have noticed, we are careful to insist a great deal on the return of awareness of being grounded after every mental practice in order to re-balance the energies. We cannot emphasize enough the importance of this very crucial point.

4

We All have a Mission

The myth of identity

One day, a man named Nasruddin saw an amazing bird land at his window, a bird that he had never seen described in any book. Nasruddin did not like the creature because it did not fit his idea of a bird. He caught it, trimmed its wings and its tail, changed its beak and filed its claws. Then contemplating his work, he said, "Ah finally, we have a bird!"

Our system of education strongly resembles this story. Does it not try to transform these 'strange birds', i.e. certain children and teachers, into exact copies that conform to an already preconceived idea?

Imagine the resentment these creatures must feel at being deprived of their individuality. It might even make some believe that the key to success is to be like everyone else. This is where traditional wisdom challenges us and says, "There is a better way than this!"

Diversity, the vital signature of life

Every tradition is rich in testimony of the many wonderful manifestations of life. Thus in the Talmud, the wise man is dazzled by the power of the Creator who molds each individual after the first man, without any one resembling the other. Likewise in the *Bhagavad Gita*, Arjuna is told to contemplate the hundreds and thousands of divine forms, so diverse in kind, so varied in form and color. And again in the New Testament, St. Paul compares the human community to a large body, wherein each one has his proper place, like the various organs of a body. This fundamental truth should bring humanity to recognize and respect differences. Yet history abounds in fanatical attempts to reduce the "Other" to a facsimile. If you refuse, it is *Shoah*, eradication.

Biology and medicine are confronted daily with the richness of life. The fact that each one of us is unique in the world makes the transplantation of organs a very delicate process, with the phenomenon of the rejection of organs, its tangible proof.

Faced with the currently sorry-state of society resulting from widespread standardization and with the threat hanging over our heads of replicating uniformity on a massive scale, it is more vital than ever for us to be open to differences.

That process of acceptance is already underway. See, for example, how we readily validate innovation that breaks down stereotypes when it serves an economic need. Open-minded people consider innovation to be the best means for overcoming this opposition to progress. In school, as well as in all walks of life, we have to be bold enough to be who we are.

Economic reality and traditional wisdom agree on one point at least; our creative genius cannot blossom unless we have confidence in and value our specificity. Rather than inflate us with pride, this search for authenticity gradually leads us to discover our proper place in the world. As Emmanuel Levinas writes, "To be free is to do that which nobody else can do in my place."

"If I am not myself, who will be?"

This question of the sage, Hillel, has come down to us through the ages. In yoga, there is a term associated with this: *swadharma*. What does this word mean? It defines our proper place in life, that which requires an intense determination to resist the primitive instinct of following the herd. Our reptilian brain does not demand more from us than to dive into routine, thus losing ourselves in the madding crowd. Hitler's mass appeal has been one terrifying example, but fortunately the destiny of humankind lies elsewhere.

The example of great men has shown that it is necessary to obey the voice of your conscience. The practice of yoga gives us the power to focus on our internal messages and to translate them in day-to-day life.

To be true to oneself is a narrow path that frightens many people. But a life lived following a road less traveled can lead to levels of high accomplishment. Teachers need to give as much emphasis to the child's creative trials and errors as they do to his right or wrong answers. All too often in the past we have favored the prowess of the parrot over that of the amazing bird.

Wise men say that each human being, from birth, possesses a secret name. This name is different for each one of us and is not necessarily the one chosen by our parents. The goal is to discover it and to allow it to manifest itself in the open.

All our common biblical names signify a direction in life and we do well to understand them. Elizabeth for example means "Be the house of God"; Michael, "Come closer to God". It is unfortunate that the sound and the significance of a name is no longer the focus of meditation for the parents who select it and for their children who carry it.

To live an intense life let us follow our own path and not necessarily that of our father and mother, our neighbors and friends. Great destinies often imply a complete break from the *great expectations* of the family, society and religious institutions.

To be yourself, let others be themselves.

Disobedience is not always what it seems. Let us not mistake the smoke for the fire. What really counts is our obedience to an inner vision, the voice of our deeper self. The great American thinker, Henry-David Thoreau, foresaw with clarity the birth of our consumer driven society. In the early nineteenth century, he warned his contemporaries against the dangers of a 'macadamized mind' where everyone is like everybody else. Educating means affording children every opportunity to express themselves freely. Surprising as it may seem, this approach is possible via very simple practices that invite children to be true to themselves and to be open to the differences in others.

EXERCISE 23—ACCEPTING OTHERS

We often propose this very easy exercise to children and beginners:

> "Raise the right-hand and turn it like the blade of a windmill ten times in one direction and ten times in the other, focusing your attention on the movement...*(pause)*...Lower the arms and feel the difference between the two shoulders, the two arms, the two hands *(pause)*. Tell me what you feel!"

Here are some of the contradictory answers we have received:

"My right arm feels warmer than my left one."

"No, mine feels cooler on the right."

"My right hand feels lighter than my left"

"How can that be? My right hand feels heavier."

"I feel a tingling in my shoulder."

"My shoulder is fine; it's my hand that is tingling!"

"I feel like my right shoulder is higher than the left."

"That's strange, I feel just the opposite, that my left is higher."

Some children, furious at seeing themselves contradicted, are ready to defend their position with their hands and fists. These reactions are truly a microcosm of ideological conflict; each one of us is convinced that what we believe is true, is valid for the whole world! The teacher often has to intervene to point out the intrinsic value of diverging answers, provided they are the sincere expression of the person having experienced them. Besides the release of physical tensions, this exercise has a marvelous effect on the atmosphere in class...and in society. Thus diversity of experience no longer rings synonymous with conflict, but with enrichment.

Roots, First of All

Recognizing the existence of silent areas in our brain, a process still largely unknown, heralds the evolution of mankind. But the investment of all our energies toward the development of the intellect may represent a major risk in our search for truth. In these times, when computers are in the process of surpassing us in the domain of mental performance, some people are disturbed, like the great cyber-technician, Marvin Minsky:

> *"A machine will end up with the intelligence of Mr. X or Y. It will take control of its own education....And a few months later, its power will be incalculable."*

And he adds a remark which needs to be heeded:

> *"We will not have a chance against this super-machine if it decides to keep us like pet animals."*

Are we going to let coming generations develop into computer, press-button baboons? This is the risk we run if we continue to teach our children to be walking encyclopedias who know all the branches of knowledge, but not their own roots.

Let us irrigate the tree of life at its base, not its leaves!

PART THREE

MASTER MIND
PERCHED ON ITS
TREE OF LIFE

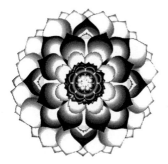

"If there is a more evolved world, why couldn't I have been born there?"

With the above caption in mind, the caricature of an under-privileged child beckons us from a billboard. Imagine that a visitor from a highly evolved galaxy comes to watch the life of our students at school. He might with good reason think of us as barbarians when he sees how we treat our children who are wedged between tables and chairs, often for eight hours a day, made to swallow subject after subject—language, mathematics, natural sciences, history, geography—without a breather.

Indeed, this state of barbarianism has already been identified by doctors under the general term 'intensive schooling'. We hear a lot of talk about respecting biological rhythms. Meanwhile, discoveries in the neurosciences have not succeed-ed in making us modify the crazy school timetables that make learning as pleasant as bonded labor. A mass of information is crammed into the student's head; no wonder the appetite for learning dwindles. Yet we continue to ignore the laws of 'diges-tion' of knowledge.

Yoga proposes that we should return to common sense in accordance with the latest research on the brain.

Educating the mind of your child

Yoga is based on a basic tenet that, far from being fixed in a defined structure from birth, the brain keeps changing throughout life. The goal of the exercises presented in Part Three is precisely to awaken the immense potential of the brain in a systematic manner in keeping with the latest science.

A striking example is Robert Sperry's work on the functioning of the two hemispheres of the brain, for which he won the Nobel Prize in 1981. For example, a patient with disconnected hemispheres can recognize an object placed in his left hand but cannot name it. Likewise, he can name an object in his right hand but is unable to describe its function. This experiment throws light on:

1. The specificity of each hemisphere.

2. The necessity of cooperation between the two halves of our brain.

Yoga offers just this, via a gamut of exercises for the left/right polarity, designed to harmonize the brain energy. Below is a classic eye exercise that allies the hemispheres.

EXERCISE 24 — POLARIZED BREATHING WITH A HELPING FINGER

Transcription of a session with a class:

"Be seated comfortably, straighten your backs and feel the soles of your feet firmly planted on the ground. Raise your hands to your head. Place your two index fingers at eye level, a few inches from your face, like this. *(The teacher demonstrates the position with her index fingers.)*

"Look at the tip of your left index finger. Breathe in deeply. Breathe out, slowly move the finger towards the left and follow its movement with your eyes without moving your head *(short pause)*.

"Now, your lungs are empty. While breathing in, bring your finger back towards the center to your starting position *(pause)*. With your lungs full, look at the tip of the right index finger and, breathing out, move the finger towards the right. Follow it with your eyes *(pause)*. Bring the finger back again to the center as you breathe in."

Repeat this exercise five times on each side, remembering to keep your eyes focused on the tip of the finger. Synchronize your breath to the movement of your fingers and eyes while keeping your head steady *(pause)*. Lower your hands and close your eyes. Observe your breathing in both nostrils.

Remarks

This exercise of polarization connects breathing and sight and exerts a powerful influence on the two brain hemispheres. It re-establishes the flow of pranic energy and allows the two sides of your head to establish a good relationship with each other. Scientific research shows that the movement of the eyes in one direction has an effect on the opposing cerebral hemisphere. This age-old yogic practice lends to this modern-day discovery an easy application. It excels in establishing the child's balance. As a bonus, it strengthens the eyes.

Responding to the subtle senses

According to yoga tradition, human beings are endowed with not just five but twenty senses. Some of you will say, "so much the better! We're richer than we thought we were." But not everyone will be convinced. So in order to show just how rich our sensory perception is, let us start with the example of a most commonplace experience, the dream:

"You are asleep in your bed and you are dreaming that you are in the mountains, in a meadow where there are cows with ringing bells. Your eyes can perceive the bright green grass and the darker color of the tall fir trees. Your ears hear the sound of the bells. You are walking through the field enjoying the delicious taste of chocolate which delights your palate. Your nostrils quiver with the scent of the fresh mountain air.

"In fact, you are in your room, at night. Even when your sense organs are disconnected from the external world, you undoubtedly have an intense sensory experience. You inhale, you taste, you see, you listen; and you, a city dweller deprived of nature, may dare in a dream, the courage to stroke the rough back of a cow. Of course, you will not deny yourself the pleasure of making small talk with the shepherd or shepherdess...From this point onwards anything can happen.

"We will leave you to dream."

Through this example it is easy to confirm that we all possess inner senses, which in yoga are called the subtle senses. They allow us to have psychic experiences independent from external stimuli. These subtle senses can also be activated in a waking state as in the case of a daydream or through deliberate visualization. In our everyday consciousness, we often program our acts so that we experience them before we actually do them. Haven't you ever 'seen' yourself boarding a train before you've even arrived at the station?

Any preparation, whether it be an exam or a meeting, is enhanced by being imagined in advance. This process can be spontaneous or intentional with the aim of facilitating the accomplishment of the previewed action. For example, a sportsman does not train himself only on the track but also in his head. The three time Olympic ski champion, Jean-Claude Killy, said that he performed the route of his descent at least a hundred times over mentally before the actual competition.

We can thus multiply by two the five senses that we normally link with our knowledge of the external world. However, according to yoga, we must add to these five senses of knowledge another set, the five senses of action: feeling, locomotion, speech, excretion and procreation. These five senses of action also have their subtle counterpart. Patrick Segal, a hemiplegic, calls himself 'a man who walks in his head." Adding all these together gives us twenty senses. This is not just a mental game of splitting hairs, so to speak, but a reality that puts us in touch with the extraordinary richness of our senses so that we may fully appreciate and enjoy them.

In our civilization, unfortunately, we educate children using no more than their external senses and even these are restricted to the audio-visual. Notice, for example, how little we use the sense of smell or taste in school teaching? But what is even more serious is the neglect of our interior senses.

The part played by the subtle senses is practically non-existent at school. We have failed to recognize them as the bridge, allowing us to relate the presentation of knowledge to its intellectual understanding.

Visualization, therefore, applies to all the senses including, of course, motricity and the mental pronunciation of words and sentences. We have verified that by putting in place as wide a range as possible of activities for all the senses, we significantly improve the capacity of children to assimilate and remember what we teach them. This, according to us, is the **key to learning how to learn.**

Each of our senses corresponds with a specific area of the brain. Thus, the visual area, for example, is found in the occipital lobe. The subtle senses do not function from the same zones as their corresponding external sense organs. Spoken language and mental repetition belong to different areas in the brain. So, we can deduce the following law: The more we **solicit** the senses (internal and external) in teaching a concept, the more the related cerebral surface grows. We should strive to have children **assimilate with the entire brain.** This will greatly improve the quality of teaching and of learning.

EXERCISE 25 — HOW TO MAKE RAPID PROGRESS IN SPELLING

This exercise should be done before a lesson in spelling. The notebooks are kept open on the table. The teacher is at the blackboard and she writes the following sentence:

"Sally has gone for a walk in the park with her dog."

The teacher asks the children to follow along with their eyes on the page in the book while she reads the phrase aloud very slowly. The teacher can point out, in passing, the double 'L' consonant in "Sally" whereas the 'L' is silent in "walk". For example, she might say, "notice how this is the first time that we are discussing the present perfect tense with the past participle of the irregular verb 'to go'." So far, no rules have been explained to the children.

Each pupil is asked to re-read the sentence mentally. There is total silence in the class. Now, ask them to shut their eyes. The teacher erases the sentence. She says to them:

"Carefully watch the light filtering through your eyelids. Relax your eyes *(pause)*. Now, behind the forehead, imagine a blackboard, with a variety of chalks in different colors. Pick the one that you like and write the sentence that I'm going to read out to you. As you do this, you may move your hand on the outside as if you were writing the sentence on a blackboard in the air."

The teacher says the sentence again, very slowly:

"Sally has gone for a walk in the park with her dog."

The students write it mentally on their inner blackboard. Most of them will also form the letters with their index fingers in the air. Now the teacher says:

"Now, re-read the sentence, keeping your eyes closed. Mentally say each word that you see inside your head. Did you remember to use a capital and lower case letters and to punctuate the end of the sentence with a period? If not, correct it!" *(pause)*

"Relax for a second, keeping your attention on the light coming through your eyelids..."

"Move your attention to the soles of your feet *(short pause)*. Slowly open your eyes and write the same sentence in your notebook." *(silence)*

The teacher writes the sentence again and the pupils compare it with their notebooks. If there is a mistake, the child is instructed to correct it in his book but also – and this is what is important – in his inner register by reproducing the correct form on his mental screen. Children will see for themselves that in this way, the number of their mistakes becomes minimal.

Remarks

Notice the *progression* of the exercise in moving from external to internal and then from internal to external. Always be careful of the transitions *(the light through the eyelids)* between the external world and the time of internalization. This exercise is most effective.

Students of yoga will recognize this as a practice of *raja yoga* applied to education.

This exercise can be adapted for use in other subjects besides spelling, as it holds the attention of children of all ages, from primary to high school level.

EXERCISE 26 — REVIEWING THE PROPERTIES OF A RECTANGLE

1. Draw a rectangle on the blackboard, for example, and write its characteristics around it.
2. The students are told to read each of the six characteristics successively, moving in a clockwise direction from one to the next and following a three-step procedure for each point:

First, mentally repeat the property.

Second, check to make sure that you understand the property illustrated.

Third, go back to the center and fix your gaze briefly on the middle point, before moving on to the next property. *(Silence in the class)*

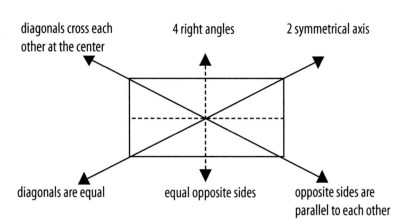

3. Eyes closed, and after having drawn a rectangle on the mental screen, the students are asked to visualize the six characteristics of the rectangle in whatever color they like, and to repeat each of them mentally. For example, the pupil says silently to himself, 'four right angles', and mentally colors the four angles in red. Next, he turns his attention back to the central core of the drawing a second time, before moving on to saying silently 'two symmetrical axis', and coloring them, and so on.

Remarks

This way of handling geometry helps a lot of children understand figures in space. This exercise of visualization is also good in learning three dimensional forms such as spheres, pyramids and cubes.

Helping children to carry through an action

In our educational system that veers heavily towards the abstract, more emphasis is given to concepts than to concrete practical application. To remedy this imbalance requires more than just a switch in text books. The brain of a child develops best when it is given an idea with a concrete example. Like the great yogi Sivananda said, "An ounce of practice has more value than ten tons of theory."

Are you familiar with Mark Rosenzweig's famous experiments using caged rats? He and his colleagues at the University of California at Berkeley placed two groups of rats of the same family in two different types of cages: the first group was in a normal cage with a view to the world outside whereas the other was in a cage which was enriched with all sorts of objects that were replaced every day.

An analysis of their brains showed definitively and clearly that the second group of rats (1) were capable of higher learning, (2) had a cerebral cortex that was thicker than the other group, (3) that the number of their neurons had increased and above all, (4) that their inter-neural connections had increased by more than 20%.

The control group, which was content to look without doing anything, had simple normal brains that could be described as mediocre, in comparison with those of the rats in the second group.

This experiment proves undoubtedly that not only sensations but also actions are nourishment for the brain.

Recommendation

Whenever possible, cultivate children's common sense and mental maturity by allowing them to take on practical responsibility for tasks in everyday life.

Endocrine storms within the child

All young people inevitably go through various intense periods of crisis as they are growing up. The passage into the age of reason (6-7 years) is one; then there is the "somersault" of puberty that upsets the child. In the olden days, we helped the child surmount this passage through rites of initiation with the object of helping them integrate their impulses into their social life. Today, we notice that children have to go through this period of maturation without any real guidance.

We interviewed a great master of yoga as well as a man of science on this topic, Swami Satyananda. He said that in India, children are introduced by their fathers to the practices of yoga from the age of seven.

Contemporary science shows us that at this age a physiological event takes place that affects the brain to a great extent: the pineal gland begins to degenerate. It is a natural phenomenon that up to the age of seven, the pineal gland is intensely active. When we watch a baby, we are amazed at the speed at which it grows, learns and develops. This early growth is orchestrated by the pineal gland. Even as its effectiveness begins little by little to diminish, the child of course continues to grow until the age of eighteen years or more, but at a slower pace.

From the moment that the pineal gland slows down its production of hormones, another gland, the pituitary, enters the scene becoming the 'leader' of the endocrines. This gradual transfer of roles, however slow, has a considerable influence on the child because it allows him to access the powerful force of natural instincts. Indeed, it is the pituitary gland that triggers the function of the sexual glands which will continue to grow in strength until they reach full maturity at the time of puberty.

Yoga stresses that these processes should be retarded naturally by slowing down the degeneration of the pineal gland. Yogis claim that this gland does not dwindle automatically and that it is possible to prolong its life through specific practices.

The young child lives in a world different from ours. We are so proud of our ability to reason but we have paid a heavy price for it: the weakening of our capacity to visualize. Children make all imagined things real and test everything they encounter as living. They will spontaneously speak to a tree, a toy or an animal. This ability in childhood is one of the most precious gifts of life. Unfortunately, very few educators know how to keep it alive beyond the realm of fairy tales. This change in the state of consciousness is sometimes reflected in the drawings of children whose inspiration changes, sometimes suddenly, within the first years of their primary education.

Today, we are witnessing sexual development in children at ever younger ages. It often disturbs the course of their studies. Occasionally, it changes the child into a "storm zone". It goes without saying that their apparent lack of interest in studies seems to be the lesser evil in comparison to the disastrous effects endocrine whirlwind has on their behavior. Imagine a twelve-year-old youngster feeling the same passionate attractions and inner conflicts as a thirty-year-old adult. How can he, at his age, endure the tornado of impulses that are unleashed within him? Often, he will release some of this pent-up violence in anger and rebellion against his family and environment, leaving parents and teachers distressed and helpless. This is undoubtedly a social phenomenon; however, the analysis by sociologists and psychologists does not go far enough, for they neglect essential physiological factors that we have just outlined.

Yoga has devised practices that give us many ways of slowing down the premature secretion of sexual hormones.

Recommendations

From the age of seven or eight, teach your children the sequence of dynamic postures, like the "Small Salutation to Work" *(Exercise 7, page 32).*

Teach them early on to simply observe their breathing in the nostrils, without changing the rhythm or the depth of the breath.

Make them practice the very gentle exercises of polarized breathing, like the alternate nostril breathing while following the sides of a triangle *(Exercise 11, page 46).*

Of utmost importance are mental images. Visualization, which children love, will naturally bring their attention to the forehead at a point which, according to the science of yoga, stimulates the pineal gland through a reflex action. Try it out for example with the practice "a chain of words" *(Exercise 17, page 66).*

According to us, these recommendations give many methods to help parents and teachers educate the younger generation at the threshold of today's world.

Massage your brain—Experience the marvelous effects of a journey of awareness through the different parts of the body.

Every action that we do, every sensation that we feel, relates to a certain area of our brain. Look at the two little creatures in Diagram 1; each one is endowed with a big head and a huge hand, where we clearly notice the thumb. Note that the thumb has played a primordial role in human evolution because it allowed us to hold tools.

Diagram 1 shows us that all the parts of the body correspond to specific zones in the brain along the Fissure of Rolando. We can roughly map out the path which is pictured here along the curve of the cranial dome if we imagine the headband of an earphone headset.

Each part of our body is represented along this line here, not according to its surface area but its neural network. For example, as we can see, the hand and the mouth take up larger zones than the leg and the trunk.

Each of our movements is directed by the part of the brain to which it corresponds.

For children it is essential to have a good awareness of their body schema. When they are immobile in relaxation and we mention one by one, each part of the body, we create in them a systematic massage of the corresponding area in the brain.

According to recent research, this type of rotation of consciousness through the bodily parts carries its effects over into everyday life, thereby helping the subject to coordinate his

DIAGRAM 1 —BRAIN MAP OF THE BODY HOMUNCULOUS

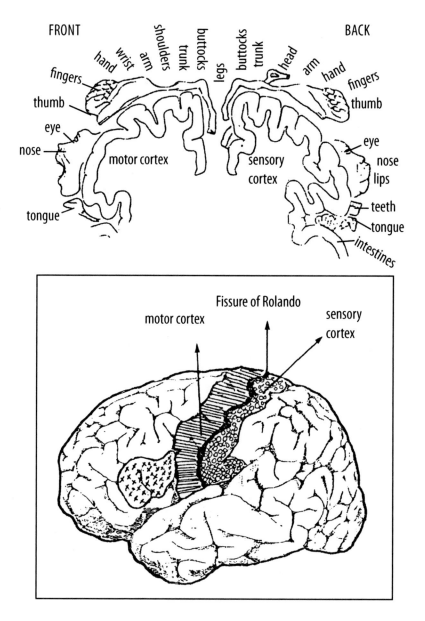

physical movements. This practice entails a spontaneous relaxation of tensions and contractions.

Transmitted through the tradition of yoga, this technique brings to light the accurate knowledge that ancient sages had of the nervous system. Without any instruments of measure, they established the location of the pathways of energy with such precision that it continues to command our admiration.

EXERCISE 27 — AN EXCURSION AROUND THE BODY ISLAND

Here is the transcription of a live session in a classroom that illustrates what we are going to try to explain. The children have all chosen their favorite image or their key phrase beforehand. They are listening to the teacher. During the rotation of consciousness through the body parts, pause for a short time between each part so that the students have the time to mentally repeat the name of the body part called out while sensing it quickly as well. This technique is based on the voice and on listening. This implies a certain rhythm in the calling out of each body part which the written transcription can only suggest but not completely render:

- "Sit in a comfortable position. Take time to feel completely at ease. You will need to sit for about ten minutes, without moving, with your eyes shut. From this moment onwards, bring your attention effortlessly to the instructions that I give you. *(pause)*

- "Listen to the sounds outside at the same time as you listen to the sounds inside the classroom. *(pause)* I will now make three small sounds which you will hear. First sound: *(crumpling of paper)*, second sound: *(clicking of a ballpoint pen)*, third sound: *(footsteps)*. Mentally name each of the

122

three sounds that you heard me make, in the same order as I made them; listen to them within yourself. *(pause)* Now, observe your breathing through your nostrils. *(pause)* You are relaxed and you are observing your silence and that of the whole class.

• Repeat your key phrase or visualize your favorite image. *(pause)* Now, become aware of your entire body once again, your contact with the chair, your feet on the floor, your hands on the table. We are going to take a journey around the body and explore it as if it were an island. We will start as usual with the thumb of the right hand. Remember to repeat mentally the name of each body part that you feel as I mention it:

Right hand, right hand thumb; second finger, third, fourth, fifth, top of the hand, palm, wrist, elbow, shoulder, right side of the chest, waist, hip, thigh, knee, calf, ankle, heel, top of the foot, sole of the foot, big toe, second, third, fourth, fifth.

Left hand, left hand thumb, second finger, third, fourth, fifth, top of the hand, palm, wrist, elbow, shoulder, left side of the chest, waist, hip, thigh, knee, calf, ankle, heel, top of the foot, sole of the foot, big toe, second, third, fourth, fifth.

The entire back of the body, spinal column, nape of the neck, scalp.

The entire front of the body, face, forehead, eyes, ears, cheeks, nose, mouth, lips, teeth, tongue, throat, chin, head and neck, chest, abdomen, lower abdomen, shin, feet.

The whole body, the whole body, the whole body.

• Become aware of your breath calm, like the waves of the sea around the island that you are. Count seven waves. *(pause)*

• Now, once again, visualize your favorite image or repeat your key phrase.

- Slowly, very slowly, gently move your fingers, then your feet, your head. Taking in a deep breath, gently open your eyes and look in front of you.

(End of the session).

Tradition

This is a very short practice session of a technique called *Yoga Nidra.*

Remarks

One must pay very close attention to the transitions, especially at the end of the practice. The return to movement should be done very slowly.

To avoid shock due to the contrast, it is recommended that a gentle manual activity, like drawing, be used at the end of the session. This should have been announced before the start of the relaxation. Notebooks and textbooks, pencils and compasses should be ready on the table before the beginning of the relaxation practice.

PART FOUR

YOGA
À LA CARTE

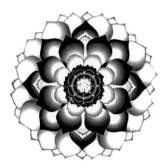

"Is yoga practice specific to India?"

No, it is to be found in all civilized traditions and at all latitudes of the globe. But what then are the criteria of an exercise that allow us to include it in the category of yoga?

- The proposed technique must be linked to the definition of yoga, which can be found in the germ of the etymology of the word yoga. The Sanskrit root *yug* is found in all Indo-European languages and has a similar meaning: thus, in English we have the word "yoke" which is used to "join" two animals together. The origin of these words goes back to the beginning of man's effort to unite his physical and mental forces.

- Yoga requires presence of mind: It is more yogic to raise the index finger with complete awareness, than to stand on your head or to sit in the lotus position while thinking of the delicious meal that you are going to have or remembering a letter you have just received.

- Yoga exercises are as diverse as people so it is more accurate to speak of yoga in a plural sense than to imagine it as a single entity. According to tradition, each practitioner should receive personalized directions from his teacher. Yoga "à la carte" is a better way, one that allows each of us to blossom to our full potential.

- Yoga pacifies the mind. A traditional image which describes this state is to think of the surface of a lake that reflects the sun's rays as broken shards of light. Working on oneself entails turning the lake of our mind into a mirror which reflects the sun's radiance. Therefore, we should never lose sight of the fact that yoga relaxes us and gives us a 'joie de vivre'.

Throughout all civilizations, we can find examples of authentic yogic methods for the education of mankind. For example, in ancient Egypt children were taught at school how to keep the spinal column perfectly erect. We know this for a fact because of the frescos which depict the postures clearly: the arms in the candlestick position, the bringing together of the shoulder blades and aligning the two shoulders and arms results in a marvelous straightening of the spine which was called the 'Djed pillar', *djed* being a term that refers for example to the uplifted stability of a tree, firmly rooted in the ground. We can also find yogic postures in the stone statues of Pre-Columbian art.

For us, yoga, an age-old science, can be marvelously adapted to children of the twenty-first century in a wide variety of situations. We will now reply to some of the most frequently asked questions of parents and teachers.

"How do you adapt yoga to the needs of my child?"

Yogic exercises described in the traditional texts, seem practically inaccessible to children. For example, in Tibetan yoga, the adept is asked to concentrate on a grain of rice or on the image of the Buddha for more than one hour. For a child whose mind craves a large variety of colors and attractive forms, a grain holds almost no interest. On the other hand, the exercise of concentration is excellent, provided it:

1. Be limited to one minute.

2. Motivates the child by proposing an immediate and interesting result. For example, after having fixed their gaze on a red circle, have them close their eyes and let them discover on the screen of the forehead, as if by magic, the after-image of the circle... in green! *(Exercise 19, page 80, The Magic Circle.)*

When it comes to the image of the Buddha, it carries with it the major disadvantage of depicting yoga as a religion rather than as the science that it is. Yogic exercises need to be shorn

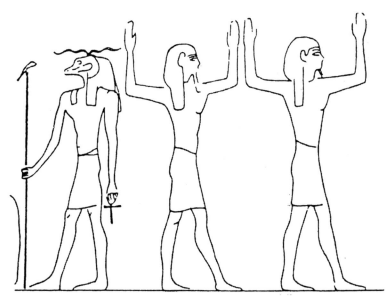

▲
The "Egyptian Walk",
with arms in the candelabra
position

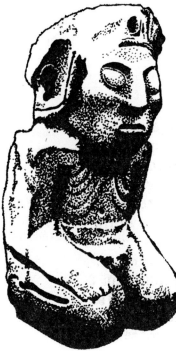

◄
The Pre-Columbian stone
statue, representing the yogic
posture 'vajrasana'

of their folkloric elements so that they become a little bit like Japanese painting whereby, with one stroke of the brush, the essential silhouette of the object is achieved. We can sum this up in two words: rigor and flexibility.

Below are some recommendations to help children benefit fully from the science of yoga:

- *Vary the exercises:* the child is a being, growing at a phenomenal pace. Thus, he craves a continual change in techniques and rejects monotony. Just as parents know that he will soon tire of a toy once the novelty has worn off, teachers need to be careful not to spoil the good effects of an exercise by doing it too often. Therefore, have in your repertory at all times *a wide variety of practices* and methods of presentation at your disposal from which to draw from in class.

- *Present the exercises as springboards towards success:* Children are much keen to the idea of self improvement, to developing attention, memory and creativity. Since yoga is a means of achieving quality education, this is an excellent reference and the best motivation for children who wish to succeed. Besides, they will very quickly realize on their own the benefits of the techniques that they practice. The exercises that we propose in this book have already helped thousands of students to concentrate better and to achieve academic excellence that they did not believe possible before.

- *Explain to your child that he is like an astronaut who is about to take off on the conquest of inner space.* Beginning to do yoga is like setting off on an exciting adventure; it is to enter into the discovery of oneself by exploring the various galaxies which populate our inner system, such as:

  The Constellation of the Body and its Smallest Recesses. Let your child, for example, leave on a mission towards that often very tense star of his system known as the solar plexus, and learn to relax it.

The Whirling Constellation of Emotions. The child-astronaut often finds himself in the middle of a storm flickering signals announcing a chaotic galaxy in full formation. What a waste of energy! It should be channeled through yoga.

The Constellation of Thoughts. To our child-astronaut, this constellation is made up of many shooting stars which distract him from contemplating that one marvelous star, the core of his inner universe, the source of all energy, all light.

Yoga allows your child not only to learn more efficiently but to replenish the powerhouse of energy which lies dormant within and which will enable him to perform at his peak. In our experience, this inner voyage from galaxy to galaxy towards the "treasure star" captivates a child's interest more than all the electronic games put together. It is a rewarding quest where the child has everything to gain. This book gives you the various stages of the voyage *(Cf. Part One: The Landmarks of Success).*

- *Take into account the morphology of the child.* We know that the cartilage and ligaments of children are much more delicate than those of adults. Thus, it is not advisable to insist on immobility for a long time in postures requiring flexing, extension and twisting. Since the growth of the spinal column is not yet complete, it is imperative to take care that it develops straight and strong. It is especially important to correct the lumbar curve. We suggest you have the children do the pivoting exercises for the pelvis. *(Cf. Part One, Chapter 3: Walk Tall!)*

- *Do not 'put the cart before the horse'.* Do not try to go too fast; yoga involves a gradual process. Following a sequence of the exercises implies fidelity to the yogic code which correctly stresses the progression from the physical plane to the mental. As for breath, it is situated exactly at the interface of these two. Indeed, our breathing interacts with the body in a myriad of physiological manifestations, but it is equally related to the mind and the expression of our emotions. We express relief with a sigh, surprise by the suspension of breath, and calm in the decrease of our diaphragmatic movement. The various stages of this progression correspond to the exercises in *Part One: The Landmarks of Success.* Do not get caught up in only one aspect of the practice. It is necessary to take into account the totality of the child's vital force in order to facilitate the complete and simultaneous blossoming of the body, emotions and intellect. Let us not confine yoga, as is so often the case, to a simple training of the physical body. Yoga, according to its authentic tradition, lies in the smooth functioning of all the many components of the personality, together. Harmony and coherence are the primary goals. Teachers and children alike must initially and above all become balanced individuals.

"And what if my child does not want to do yoga?"

Parents and teachers are always putting this question to us. We invariably start off our reply by reiterating that yoga should never become an unpleasant duty, forcibly imposed on a child. Let us keep in mind that yoga is associated with good mood and relaxation. How can you expect a child to learn to breathe correctly in the stifling environment of constraint or when it is perceived as a punishment?

"Your grades are unsatisfactory...

"Instead of watching the tennis match that you like on television, you will go to your room and do an hour of yoga!" Aggressive words like these prevent yoga from being a pleasurable experience and should be absolutely proscribed.

The child's attitude towards yoga depends largely on yours.

If you are convinced of the positive effects of yoga through first hand experience, you will be able to present it in an intelligent and pleasant manner to the child. It is necessary that he understand and feel the need for the exercises that you are proposing to him. A good way is to involve him in an experiment on himself and then to ask him whether the experiment has been successful. Does he feel better within? Is he better focused, calmer?

"And if my child persists in his refusal to do yoga?"

Well, let him be. Let him get involved in other things. We are not all made to like the same things. Yoga will get the child nowhere if his heart is not in it. To practice yoga under duress makes no sense, because one cannot achieve the union of energies in someone through force.

For the teacher who is trying to introduce yoga in the class, several cases may arise, such as:

The case of **the isolated child** who opposes yoga by his inertia in not doing any of the movements. This is a way of expressing his refusal. As long as he does not disturb the class, the teacher can easily let him be, without embarrassing him by requiring him to publicly justify his attitude. The teacher can possibly question him after the course, in private. Sometimes a pupil will come up on his own after class and tell the teacher that he has pain in his back or shoulder or has a headache. There was a case when one pupil who, being slightly deaf, did not want to close his eyes because he followed the directions by reading the lips of the teacher. It can also happen that one or more pupils in a group become defensive out of shyness or due to a prejudice against yoga. In such circumstances, you must be patient and wait. Often the prejudice disappears. If not, one can ask the child to study his lesson in silence while the others do the exercise.

Two cases of spoilsports:

The Giggler. This reaction is most prevalent at the beginning of the year, when students are becoming acquainted with exercises that they have never done and which appear really weird to them, especially coming from teachers in academic disciplines. When first challenged by a giggler, many fellow teachers have become discouraged, in spite of their enthusiasm to introduce yoga in their classrooms. More often than not, we are wrong to reprimand students harshly for laughing without understanding that this sometimes comes as a spontaneous response on the child's part to a surprise. Laughter is an excellent means for the child to release tensions. The expression 'a burst of laughter' means that the lungs are emptied fully and abruptly and that the person is 'joking'. It is an excellent opportunity to show the children that the reflex of laughter occurs when the lungs are full and the breath is suspended. Usually, the children will get over the surprise effect and begin to understand the value of these exercises. When this happens, the giggling disappears.

The professional disrupter. He is often a problem child. There are hyper-active children in our classes. The fact is very well known today. These children seem to refuse any sort of discipline. Whereas some problem children end up loving the exercises which calm them, other cases remain unresponsive and rebellious. These we will sometimes send out of the classroom to complete a task, so that the other children can benefit from the atmosphere of silence and calm which they enjoy a great deal.

It is obvious that children are not always interested in doing yoga. It is up to the teacher to sense whether the moment is opportune. There is an element of intuition involved in good judgment. However, one thing is certain: Our attitude as teachers is a key element with regard to whether the disrupter will prevail.

"My child has trouble doing his homework and concentrating."

For example, one mother tells us, "Johnny cannot concentrate on his homework... it is not that he doesn't try. But, you know, we live in a small apartment right in the center of town where there is a lot of street noise around. Then he complains that his two year old sister is crying all the time and getting into everything. His father doesn't help matters either. As soon as he gets home from work, he turns on the television to relax. How can I blame him? The other day, Johnny was so fed up with it all that he shut himself up in the closet and put balls of cotton wool in his ears so that he could memorize his poetry assignment."

This kind of situation occurs frequently. At home after school, when a child has homework to do, he often faces difficult choices. His intention to work conflicts with the multiple temptations that vie for his attention, such as the radio, television, snacks, telephone, computer, video games and so on. When he finally settles down to do his homework, it is important that he should know how to focus his attention on the task. He must make a conscious effort to concentrate on one thing. How can he learn to put the various surrounding stimuli on hold?

The capacity to withdraw yourself from your environment is not innate. We teach it to ourselves and gradually develop it like a muscle. We could quote dozens of examples here of children who, thanks to the techniques of yoga proposed in this book, finally succeeded in concentrating perfectly on their studies, even in the midst of a myriad of distractions.

If there is one word that withstands time in its ability to mobilize crowds and the media, it is 'freedom' —the freedom of enterprise, the freedom of the press, the freedom of women, and the freedom of thought. Don't all these forms of freedom assume that the individual is free? And isn't concentration an essential aspect of our individual freedom? The person who cannot collect the scattered flow of his attention in the face of agitation and noise is not really free. In order to speak of freedom, in full knowledge of the facts, in order to remain connected to what is going on, don't we also need to know how to withdraw at will from the undesirable audiovisual stimuli we are slave to?

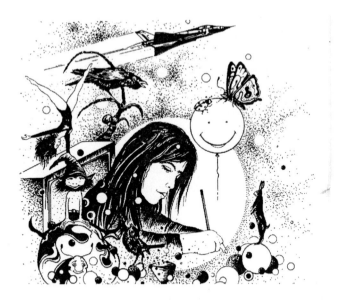

The child must learn to isolate himself in a bubble of silence in the middle of surrounding disturbances.

Recommendations

Test your own ability to withdraw yourself from surrounding disturbances. Go to a noisy cafe with a piece of work you have to complete. Initially, listen attentively to all the noise around you while remaining neutral to it. Now, select a noise, even an intermittent one, and listen to it with constant attention. If you have a watch with a second hand, follow it for one minute. Once this time has lapsed, you can set about your task with focused attention. Now help your child to focus using what you have learned.

Help your child focus attention on homework — try using some of these exercises.

Exercise 11. Alternate Breathing: The Triangle
Exercise 14. Closing the Doors
Exercise 16. The Point and the Circle

Exercise 18. The Game of Listening and Silence
Exercise 19. The Magic Circle

"My child is sad and lacks self-confidence."

"My fourteen year old daughter, Pamela, has stopped smiling. If she does let go the slightest nervous laugh, it sounds more like a sob than a real outburst of joy. Nothing seems to matter to her; she has lost her enthusiasm. She sits despondently for hours in an armchair and does nothing. She replies to our concern rhetorically with, 'What's the point of working hard in order to get ahead? In any case, I'll never get good enough grades, and besides, even if I did, the job market is completely saturated. There are hundreds of candidates for every single job and one thing is sure, the person who's going to get chosen isn't me.' Pamela does not seem to believe in anything any more and least of all in herself. Nevertheless, I told her time and again that she's not doing anything to make herself look better, that she is losing her beauty and charm and that she should be trying everything to pull herself together again, but she won't."

Like Pamela, sadness in young people is almost always accompanied by a negative self image, a sense of failure and uselessness. But the darkness which settles inside us needs nourishment in order to thrive and carry on its undermining work. What does it feed on? Negative thoughts that we ruminate incessantly, like Pamela in her armchair: "I'll never get good enough grades. Even if I did, the job market is completely saturated. The person who's going to get chosen isn't me." Gaining momentum through repetition, these pessimistic thoughts end up creating huge black clouds in our inner space which are then reflected on the outside.

In addition, Pamela's mother adds insult to injury when she tells her: "She's not doing anything to make herself look better...she is losing her beauty and charm...she should...pull herself together again."

How should we react in this situation? We should begin

by starving the "melancholy monarch" seated on the throne of our personality by feeding him positive thoughts which will replace the negative ones.

Be a positive pole. Instead of pushing the child deeper into a negative self-image by unpleasant remarks, emphasize the slightest glimmer of hope that shines on the horizon. By your attitude and words, inject a large dose of positive thoughts into the atmosphere, both at home and at school. For more on this subject, read the section in Part One, Chapter 2 entitled "*When confidence generates confidence*".

Be objective. Encourage your child as often as possible to observe recurring negative thoughts. Look back in the book to *Part Two, Exercise 21—The Witness.* Have your child write down some of the dark thoughts that haunt him. In the same way, also have him write down the opposite, positive formulation of the same thought.

In Pamela's case, she would write down: "I'll get better and better grades." She would then repeat this positive statement three times mentally.

Repeat a positive key phrase. This is above all, the most powerful antidote against negative thoughts. Teach your child to repeat regularly a positive key phrase of his own choice, so that he can positively nourish his self image. For more about this, read *The key phrase that transforms you (Part One, Chapter 2).*

How do you go about choosing a key phrase? First of all, eliminate the negative, so that, for example, instead of saying "I'm not sick any more" you choose "Everyday I'm getting better and better". A good method to narrow down your phrase is to list your principal negative thoughts next to their opposite, positive formulations. From these you will devise one short, positive sentence which summarizes them.

Always keep in mind that positive is stronger than negative; as soon as the dawn breaks, darkness vanishes. Therefore teach your child to take time during the day, especially when he is waking up in the morning and before he falls asleep at night, to repeat his key phrase calmly. These positive moments will lighten the dark sky and little by little the clouds will vanish.

Another very useful technique which reinforces this idea is *Exercise 15—The wind that chases the clouds (Part One: Chapter 6)*. The child who is sad should not lower his arms in discouragement. Help him to raise them up towards the sky, while breathing in and out as correctly and as fully as possible.

When a child feels that the world is closing in on him from all sides, teach him to open his 'house' and to fill it with fresh air! Towards this end, we suggest the following practices:

Exercise 4.   Cleaning House

Exercise 8.   The Candelabra

Exercise 10. Complete Respiration

Help free your child from dark thoughts: have him draw and color mandalas. Read about these again in *Part Two: Chapter 3*.

Depression is often the result of a loss of direction in life. To help your child find meaning in life and work towards an ideal, consult *Part Two, Chapter 4*.

"My child is tired and frazzled."

This child seems to be suffering from nervous fatigue. As teachers we are also very concerned by this syndrome which we frequently observe among children in school.

First, is it possible to identify the source of the syndrome? Is this chronic tiredness due to the process of growing up? Perhaps it arises from an unsavory relationship? Friendship plays an important role in the life of a child. It is possible that he is tense because of a bad relationship with one of his classmates. Or the problem may stem from a misunderstanding between him and his teacher or the subject being taught. Whatever the source, his tiredness is a sign that he is worried and anxious and his poor morale is sapping his energy.

There are things that can be done at the teacher and school level, but action can also be taken directly in regards to the child himself. Parents and teachers need to become aware of the quality of the child's sleep and to make sure that he has a proper dietary intake. In particular, the consumption of stimulating drinks such as tea, coffee, coke, and all other sugared liquids and sodas should be discouraged.

A good healthy diet should include ample amounts of vegetable juices, fresh fruits, dairy products and fish, with confectioneries and meats in lesser quantity. Let us not forget dried beans and vegetables as well as whole grain cereals which are so invaluable. In the olden days, some Scottish students, too poor to pay for the grand meals of Oxford and Cambridge, would each arrive at university carrying a large bag of oatmeal on their backs. For want of better means, they would have porridge for the entire year. How much of their success can be credited to this frugal regime? (In any case, the story holds that these valiant young people obtained their diplomas with flying colors!)

To fight against nervous fatigue, the following exercises are particularly recommended:

Exercise 4.   Cleaning House

Exercise 8.   The Candelabra

Exercise 10.   Complete Respiration

Exercise 12.   Short Salutation to Rest

Exercise 14.   Closing the Doors

Exercise 27.   An Excursion Around the Body Island

Here is a story of what happened when a classroom became a dormitory.

Once when I criticized my ninth graders for slouching over their desks, they replied that they were tired due to lack of sleep. So I asked them why they had gone to bed so late. Was it because of television? No, they told me. It wasn't because they'd been up very late. In fact, most of them had gone to bed relatively early but they had remained awake for a long time, restless and open-eyed, until they finally managed to fall asleep. Alarmed by what I had just heard, I broadened my investigation and discovered that almost half of the students I spoke to, regardless of age, had difficulty falling asleep. Are there yoga practices to help them?

We recognize lack of sleep to be a very widespread problem among young people. Moreover, many of those concerned are 'early sleepers'; some are even very well behaved children who do not watch television. Nevertheless, they can all be classified as "late night insomniacs". This in itself is alarming, but we must begin to worry when quite sincere students tell us that they have an easy solution to the problem—a medicine that their parents administer to them! The practice of yoga teaches us that there are natural solutions which work well most of the time.

Let's begin by using a simple breathing method, based on awareness:

EXERCISE FOR FALLING ASLEEP QUICKLY

You need to be familiar with complete breathing, the description of which is found in *Part One: Chapter 4, "Breath is life"*.

- **Breathe in for 3 seconds** while following the order of the 3 stages of respiration.

- **Hold the breath for 2 seconds.**

- **Breathe out for 5 seconds.**
  This constitutes one round.

Repeat this exercise 10 times.

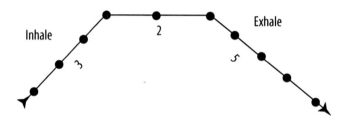

141

Furthermore, let us inculcate in young people the habit of cleansing their minds before going to sleep. Lying down on their back and relaxing deeply before falling asleep provides a rejuvenating sleep. There is nothing like a promenade through the island of the body, followed by *Yoga Nidra* (Exercise 27: An Excursion Around the Body Island) for clearing the mind of the images of war and horror that are shown to it, far too often and without reason, on TV.

Recommended Exercises

Exercise 11. Alternate Breathing: the Triangle

Exercise 24. Polarized Breathing

Exercise 27. An Excursion Around the Body Island

"My child is scared."

"I have a 13 year old son who is a good student… until it comes time for him to take a test. Then, he just goes blank and no longer seems to be himself. He panics so much that he gets bad marks. Some of his teachers realize this but not all of them. Right now my child is completely beside himself because one teacher has accused him of getting help on his homework. There is a huge difference between my son's poor test results in class and the quality of the homework assignments which he turns in, after having completed them peacefully in his room. Whenever exam time draws near, he is sick several days in advance. What can be done to help him?"

Sooner or later, all of us experience that fear which churns up the insides. It may come on the eve of a big interview or just before an important contest. Actors are such well-known victims of this that they have dubbed the phenomenon "stage-fright". Many students seem to be defenseless against it, whereas many of their teachers and professors know the very same feeling.

We have questioned students of all ages to find out what they experience before a test. The majority answer that they feel "scared" and this expressed fear is manifest in many different

142

ways, depending on the child:

"I have a tummy ache…"

"I feel sick to my stomach…"

"I can't help trembling…"

"I break out in a cold sweat…"

"It feels like something is pounding in my head…";

"Even when I know the answer, I can't seem to find the right words…".

In short, anxiety is spreading its poisonous tentacles. But what can be done to break free from its grasp?

Once again, the immediate response to this kind of distress is full breathing. The simple sound of our own breathing can sometimes be enough to bring us back to the safety of our real home, the body. This does not mean that all of the symptoms of fear will disappear, but simply by observing them, we can already lessen their power over us.

Next, remember a successful moment in your life when you have managed to overcome an obstacle. Remember the joy that you felt at the time in this accomplishment. Keeping this sense of joy alive within you, evoke the image of a sun that sheds light on your ideas at the same time as it fills you with self-confidence.

Finish with an exercise of visual or auditory concentration, and get back to work!

Recommended Exercises

Exercise 5.   The Wood Cutter

Exercise 9.   Conscious Breathing

Exercise 10. Complete Respiration

Exercise 15. The Wind that Chases the Clouds

Exercise 21. The Witness

"My child has difficulty learning his lessons."

This problem is twofold —

1. Memory

The child's difficulty may be due to **lack of memory**. It may be that this invaluable faculty of "memorizing" which endows his mind with the ability to retain and remember lessons, is not particularly brilliant. If the inadequacy is congenital, there is not much that can be done except to make note of it. However we can recommend that the child practise those exercises which will help him to develop his attention skills, both visual and listening, such as the following:

Exercise 17.   A Chain of Words
Exercise 18.   A Game of Listening and Silence
Exercise 19.   The Magic Circle
Exercise 22.   The Mandala of Associations

2. Organization

The other aspect of this difficulty may be caused by a **lack of organization**. This happens when the child is unable to place things and concepts in their proper order and sequence. We can try to teach the child how to study a lesson by taking notes. Ordinary note taking makes use of a linear sequence in outline form. We are taught to align sentences one after the other in a vertical schema which seems to us to be innate and logical. But the disorganized child may not have the same perception as we do.

There can be another way. As well acquainted as we are with the effectiveness of a circular or nuclear presentation of information, why not apply it when we set out the contents of a lesson on the blackboard? The students will show much more zeal and ease in the memorization of it using this method of presentation. It very likely corresponds to the way in which associations are made inside the brain. This method of presentation greatly assists the retention of knowledge.

You will want to refer back to Part Two, Chapter 3: Mandala, a Guiding Force as Old as the World.

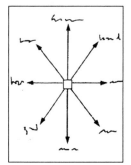

| The regular way of taking notes | Taking notes using the Mandala |

Conclusion

Teaching Teachers the Essential

Teaching education should include introductory courses in Eastern as well as Western pedagogy. Occidental practices can help teachers develop self-confidence and inner calm, and they can act as springboards to enhanced relationships with others. Teaching requires good communication skills. The art of public speaking that politicians and actors learn so assiduously in special schools also needs to be taught in our teacher training programs.

But fine tuning our body language and speech as actors do, with special emphasis placed on our presentations, misses the essential point of teaching, which is to educate the mind. The body is only one part of the human being. In it is reflected a vast territory invisible to the eyes. Any wise man will tell you that, at the core, we are all raging volcanoes whose manifestations are well-known: anger, violence, and the full range of passion and emotions, whether sadness, joy, doubt or anguish.

Our newspapers, radios and television bring to us each day echoes of this exploding "human volcano".

Political and religious systems have striven to contain or take advantage of this explosive force, to no avail. Repression and exploitation never pay off in the long run. History has shown us this, time and again. Yet the failure of our institutions to heed these lessons from the past is especially clear in regards to schools.

All powerful, except within himself, man remains "ill-bred".

Animals react to situations that they are involved in. They eat, they drink, they sleep and they reproduce, all in one body. Like us, they feel insecure and they also love. The only difference, which distinguishes them from man, is man's ability to distance himself from his instinctive reactions. Were he to lose this faculty – as we see happening in many people today – man is no more than an animal in human form. Is this where humanity is heading? If so, we may no longer speak of evolution and civilization.

But we believe that there are ways to resist this trend. Traditional wisdom offers us techniques which encourage another way of living. Teachers can knowingly take advantage of these by initially trying them on themselves and later by teaching them to their students. This is precisely the role of the teacher: To preserve and transmit our human heritage.

"Human history becomes more and more a race between education and catastrophe."

H. G. Wells (1866-1946)

These words sound all the more prophetic to us today at the beginning of the third millennium, as man's technological powers increase.

The quality of teaching must become the prime concern for our societies. We need our teachers to show children at school how to erase from their minds the seeds of violence, hatred and fanaticism. This is possible; wisdom is learning from experience.

Alchemy, the transformer of savage instincts, derives its strength in primal truths. These are brought to the surface by higher intuition that pushes us upwards to noble feelings.

How strangely beautiful it is that our teaching can take advantage of very simple, everyday experiences at every stage of life!

"I know that I am here...I feel that I am breathing... I notice tension in my back, my shoulders, my chest. I let it go... I feel revived. I am aware of others."

Today, one of the fundamental needs of the human race is to develop an awareness of our planet and an understanding that we must take time, each one of us, to live each day fully: this is the highest education. In these fleeting moments, short as they may be, we suddenly remember that we are *Citizens of the Cosmos*. Let us not run the risk with our children of allowing them to forget that they, also, are *That*. *"Tat wa asi."*

APPENDIX

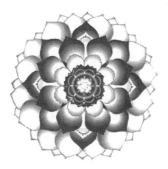

Some Western psychological techniques compared to the stages of Patanjali's Eight-fold Path. (The diagram is simplified for clarity)

Yama	Niyama	Asana	Pranayama	Pratyahara	Dharana	Dhyana	Samadhi
Relations with Others Techniques of Communication and Human Relations	Personal Hygiene All Techniques of Purification	Postures Light Gymnastics	Conscious Breath All Techniques of Conscious Respiration	Sensory Withdrawal All Techniques of Sensory Relaxation	Concentration All Techniques that develop Concentration	Meditation All states of Serenity	Illumination Self - Realization
Transactional Analysis		Alexander Eutonie Method		Alpha Methods	Vittoz Method	Prayer	
Carnegie Method	Dietary Hygiene			Biofeedback	Mind Management	Transcendental Meditation	
Massage Techniques	Dietetics	Stretching	Rebirth	Sophrology	Dream Analysis	Transpersonal Psychology	Ecstasy Enstase Satori Samadhi
Relational Assistance	Coue Method	Meziere Method	Hesychasme	Lozanov Method of Suggestopedia	Spiritual Exercises by Ignatius of Loyola	Psychedelism	
Gordon Method	Do In	Method of Noro	Bioenergy	Sensory Isolation	Mental Imagery	Out of Body Experiences	
Neuro-linguistic Programming	Dynamic Relaxation	Reeducation in Global Posturing		Chanting	Silva Mind Control	----- N.D.E.	
				Music Therapy			

Index of Exercises

Lightning Source UK Ltd.
Milton Keynes UK
UKOW050206211011

180679UK00001B/4/P

9 782905 892195